AIR FRYER RECIPES

Low Carb, Healthy and Easy to Make Air Fryer Recipes
(Delicious Recipes for Any Taste and Occasion)

Michael Osterhout

Published by Alex Howard

© Michael Osterhout

All Rights Reserved

Air Fryer Recipes: Low Carb, Healthy and Easy to Make Air Fryer Recipes (Delicious Recipes for Any Taste and Occasion)

ISBN 978-1-989891-82-7

All rights reserved. No part of this guide may be reproduced in any form without permission in writing from the publisher except in the case of brief quotations embodied in critical articles or reviews.

Legal & Disclaimer

The information contained in this book is not designed to replace or take the place of any form of medicine or professional medical advice. The information in this book has been provided for educational and entertainment purposes only.

The information contained in this book has been compiled from sources deemed reliable, and it is accurate to the best of the Author's knowledge; however, the Author cannot guarantee its accuracy and validity and cannot be held liable for any errors or omissions. Changes are periodically made to this book. You must consult your doctor or get professional medical advice before using any of the suggested remedies, techniques, or information in this book.

Table of Contents

Part 1 1
Introduction 2
RECIPES 15
Blooming Onion 15
Fried Chicken 17
Hot Wings 18
Coconut Shrimp 19
Roast Turkey Breast 20
Cherry Pie 21
Mac and Cheese 22
Country Fried Steak 23
General Tso Chicken 26
Brie Stuffed Puff Pastry 28
Corned Beef and Cabbage Egg Rolls 29
Clams oreganata 30
Roast Pork Loin with Red Potatoes 32
Fish Taco 33
Conclusion 35
Part 2 36
Introduction 37
A Brief Short History Of The Air Fryer 38
Uses Of The Air Fryer 38
How To Take Care Of Your Air Fryer 39
How To Use The Air Fyer Even On Diets 40
Not Your Ordinary Sweet Potato Fries 42
Special Baked Potato 43

Breakfast Cinnamon Rolls	44
Breakfast Hotdog Sandwich	45
Fish Sandwich	46
Meaty Beef Breakfast Empanada	47
Air-Fried Cereal	47
Breakfast Spanish Eggs with Chorizo	48
Easy Air-Fried Granola Bar	50
Classic Lemon Scone	52
Air-Fried Egg Casserole Recipe	54
Low Carb Cheesy Quiche Pepper Recipe	54
Bacon Bagels with Sesame Seeds	55
Keto Pork Sausage Casserole	57
Breakfast Lemon Muffins with Poppy Seeds	58
Low Carb Breakfast Sausage and Egg	59
Air-Fried Sweet Brownie Muffins	60
Hot Egg and Bacon Breakfast	61
Low Carb Avocado Bacon Muffins	62
Keto Cheddar Chive Ham Cups	63
Sweet Cinnamon Donut Muffins	64
Sausage and Maple Pancake Cups	65
Maple and Peanut Muffins	66
Cheesy Sausage Pie Recipe	67
Breakfast Cardamom Pumpkin Donut	68
French Toasts with a Twist	69
Fully Loaded Muffins	71
Crispy and Savory Bacon Frittata Muffins	72
Low Carb Bacon Frittata	73

Cheesy Bacon Zucchini Bread 73
Chicken Breakfast Burrito 74
Lunch Recipes 76
Cheesy Chicken Taquitos 76
Beef Tortilla Crunch-Wrap Recipe 76
Hot Chix 77
Bourbon Bacon Burger 79
All Time Favourite Turkey 80
Crunchy Avocado Fries 81
Crispy Fried Pickles 82
Air-Fried Garlic Parmesan Chicken 82
Air-Fried Cheesy Tortellini 83
Crunchy Breaded Pork Chops 84
Air-Fried Tandoori Chicken Recipe 85
Air-Fried Fish Fillets with Lemon 86
Air-Fried Sumptuous Turkey Breasts 88
My Version of Air-Fried Chicken Wings 88
Brussels Sprouts with a Twist 89
Air-Fried Healthy Fish Sticks 90
Air-fried Tasty Chicken Recipe 92
Chicken with Broccoli Zucchini Plates 93
Ham and Cheese Turnover 95
Air-Fried Cheesy Hot Dogs Bacon Wraps 97
Crunchy Tofu and Green Salad 97
Low Carb Meatballs with Guacamole 99
Keto Basil and Pepper Pizza 100
Hot and Spicy Bacon Pops 101

- Keto Personal Pizza 102
- Special Grilled Ham and Cheese Sandwich 102
- Meaty Keto Pizza 104
- Chicken Wings Different Way 105
- Air-Fried Sweet and Spicy Chicken Drummettes 106
- Keto Spiced BBQ Chicken Wings 107
- Dinner Recipes 108
- Air-Fried Italian Meatball 108
- Air-Fried Vegan Potatoes 109
- Honey Sriracha Hot Chicken Wings 110
- Healthy Fully Loaded Quinoa Burgers 111
- Southern Style Fried Pork Chops 112
- Juicy and Tender Chicken Recipe in your Air Fryer 113
- My Version of Chicken Nuggets 115
- Lemon and Ginger Chicken Recipe 115
- Buffalo-Style Cauliflower Recipe 117
- Fresh Salmon in Cajun Seasoning 118
- Healthy Friendly Orange Tangy Tofu 119
- Seasoned Fresh Fried Catfish 120
- Dinner Seasoned Shrimp with Special Sauce 120
- Ground Beef Taco with Fried Egg Rolls 122
- Creamy Mushroom Plate 123
- Cheesy Air-Fried Eggplant 124
- Spiced Turkey Taco Recipe 125
- Creamy Beef Plate Recipe 126
- Creamy Tuna Plate Recipe 127
- Cheesy Pork Rinds Recipe 128

Cheesy Burger Bacon Recipe	130
Air-Fried Nacho Chicken Recipe	132
Hot and Spicy Chicken Pops	133
Keto Italian Meatballs	134
Low Carb Pork Pie Recipe	135
Beef Chilli Peppers	135
Creamy and Cheesy Spinach Pork Roll	136
Keto Meaty Bacon Wraps	137
Keto Baked Ham and Cheese	138
Keto Bacon Cheese Bomb	139
Bread and Brie Beef	140
Beefy Bacon Stuffed Bell Peppers	141
Mozzarella Bacon Keto Meatballs	142
Cheesy Chorizo Keto Meatballs	143
Pepper and Sausage Italian Meatballs Recipe	144
Baked Italian Egg and Chicken	145
Desserts, Snacks And Appetizers	147
Chocolate and Banana Sandwich	147
My Version of Molten Lava Cake	148
Heart-Shaped Cookies	149
Sweet Dough Dippers with Chocolate Sauce	149
Air-Fried Classic Apple Pie	151
Classic Chocolate Cake in an Air-Fryer	153
Air-Fried Chocolate Frosting	153
Quick and Easy Churro Donut	154
Special Butter Cake	155
Air-Fried Jalapeno Bites	156

- Classic Snack Donuts 157
- Easy Apple Chips 157
- Special Sweet Potato Tots Snacks 158
- Pepperoni Pizza in Whole Wheat Pita Bread 160
- All-Time Favorite Banana Bread 160
- Air-Fried Keto Avocado Fries 161
- Low Carb Dessert Pudding 163
- Yummy Cream Cheesecake with Vanilla 163
- Keto Crispy Bacon Burger 164
- Healthy Snack Bars 165
- Guacamole Different Ways 166
- Mozzarella Pizza Chips 166
- Low Carb Beef Taco Tartlets 167
- Air-Fried Corndog Muffins 169
- Homemade BLT Dip 170
- Keto Crispy Onion Rings with Sauce 171
- Healthy Keto Beet Chips 172
- Cinnamon Apple Chips with Yogurt Almond Dip 173
- Super Healthy Kale Chips 173
- Air-Fried Pretzel Recipe 174
- Movie Cheesy Popcorn Puffs 175
- Crunchy Cheesy Broccoli Snack 176
- Air-Fried Mushroom Fries 177
- Air-Fried Healthy Pesto Keto Crackers 178
- Low Carb Chia Seeds Crackers 180
- Air-Fried Spiced Deviled Eggs with Bacon 182
- Keto Double Cheeseburger 183

Chia Seed Butter Snack 183
Keto Blueberry Lime Cake 185
Air-Fried Strawberry Shortcakes 187

Part 1

Introduction

I want to thank you and congratulate you for downloading this book.

Air fryers use Rapid Air Technology to cook any type of food that you would otherwise dunk in deep fat. This new technology works by circulating air to high degrees, up to 200C, to "fry" foods such as fish, chips, pastries, chicken, and more. This Rapid Air Technology is bringing in a new era of cooking appliances and a new generation of cooking methods altogether. Air fryers render foods perfectly browned and crisp with less fat–up to 80 percent less, as compared to traditional cooking methods.

Thanks again for downloading this book, I hope you enjoy it!

What is an Air Fryer?

Air fryers are all the rage in cooking. Have you seen one of the many advertisements and wondered,"How does an air fryer work?"Are you curious about the health of an air fryer? Worry no more! You have landed on the right path to answer all of your air frying questions.

Air is new oil. Ifthe term"air fryer"sounds like a lot of hot air, your speculations are exactly right! An air fryer is simply a revolutionized kitchen appliance for cooking food through the circulation of superheated air.

How Does an Air Fryer Work?

Air fryers use Rapid Air Technology to cook any type of food that you would otherwise dunk in deep fat. This new technology works by circulating air to high degrees, up to 200C, to "fry" foods such as fish, chips, pastries, chicken, and more. This Rapid Air Technology is bringing in a new era of cooking appliances and a new generation of cooking methods altogether. Air fryers render foods perfectly browned and crisp with less fat–up to 80 percent less, as compared to traditional cooking methods

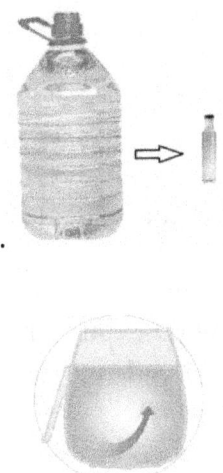

Healthy and User-Friendly

An air fryer's cooking chamber radiates heat from a heating element close to the food, thus cooking it more efficiently and appropriately. The exhaust fan located above the cooking chamber helps to provide the required airflow from the underside. This allows the heated air to constantly pass through the food. Consequently, every part of the food receives the same heating temperature. Using only a fan and grill helps the air fryer to blast hot air at a high speed, achieving the healthy qualities that you will undoubtedly notice when eating air fried food. It is a simple yet innovative method of cooking.

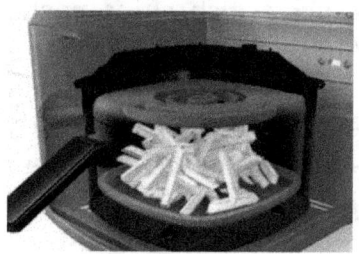

Similar to a rice cooker, an air fryer has a wide removable tray. It serves up a hot, crisp meal within 12 minutes. Though it may seem"fried"because of the crispy quality, the food cooked in an air fryer is actually healthier and reduced in calories. Philips CEO Pieter Nota said,"At Philips, we develop advanced solutions that help contribute to people's health and well-being."Anything you can think of, from chicken to chips to fish can be made healthier in an air fryer because its cooking method requires very little fat. For instance, a batch of chips only calls for half a spoonful of oil and 12 minutes to serve perfectly crispy potatoes.

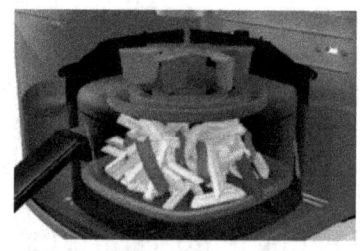

Similarly, an air fryer will give you hamburgers, steaks, and French fries in just a few minutes. You'll be amazed, but in just 25 minutes, you can bake an entire cake in an air fryer!

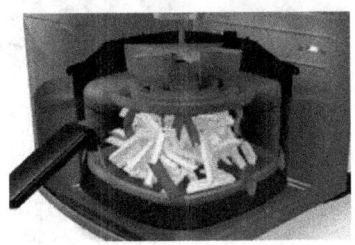

The exhaust system controls the temperature that is increased by internal pressure and emits extra air as needed to cook the food. The extra air is thoroughly filtered before being released, thus being better to the environment. Air fryers are both user and environment-friendly–harmless and odorless!

Cooling System

Do not be afraid of the superheated air that is used to cook food in an air fryer. Each comes with its own cooling system, including a fan mounted on a motor axis to control the internal temperature. This fan ensures that the environment inside the air fryer stays clean and healthy. The cooling system allows fresh air to pass through the filters and proceed to the bottom of the fryer. Allowing the passage of fresh air from top to bottom helps the air fryer to cool its internal parts.

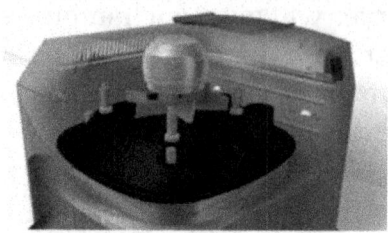

What is air frying?

The air fryer's benefits are endless. It helps users who are nervous when using a traditional chip pan and protects them from fire or burning. Its cooling systems and controlled temperature allow it to protect itself. Better tasting food, healthier meals, friendlier to the environment–we could go on and on. Try ad air fryer for yourself and discover even more benefits!

Air fryer Brief History

Air fryers were first launched in Australia and Europe in 2010, followed by North America and Japan. Today, they are a staple of the modern kitchen. The Japanese use air fryers for making fried prawns, in the Netherlands and the UK, this gadget is used for cooking chips. Americans prepare chicken wings in their air fryers. Indians use them for making samosa.

FAQ's for Air Fryer

1.   Can we cook different varieties of food in an air fryer?

Answer- Yes, you can easily cook different varieties of food in an air fryer. One of the best things about cooking food in an air fryer is that it is healthy and free from oil. Items such as meat, potatoes, poultry and French fries can be easily cooked. Apart from these items you can also bake brownies and grill different vegetables.

2. **What is the input power range of an air fryer?**
Answer- For the European market the input power range is 220 v and for USA market it is 110 v.

3. **How much time an air fryer takes to cook frozen foods?**
Answer- One of the best things to do while cooking frozen food in an air fryer is to use the knob as per the food that you are cooking. It normally takes some more time to cook frozen foods as compared to other food items.

4. **How much food can be cooked at a time in an air fryer?**
Answer- It all depends on the capacity of the air fryer. Most of the air fryers come with 500g of capacity and you can also see a"max"mark on the basket of the air fryer which means that the air fryer can be filled up to this mark.

5. **Is there any specific type of oil required for air fryer?**
Answer- No, there is no special oil which is required for cooking in an air fryer. You can us any type of oil such as olive oil, peanut oil, sunflower oil and even butter spray.

6. **Can we add more ingredients while the food is getting cooked in an air fryer?**
Answer-Yes, you can add more ingredients while the food is getting cooked in an air fryer but make sure to add the ingredients immediately otherwise the heat loss may lead to more time consumption for cooking the food.

7. **Is it possible to use baking paper or aluminum foil in an air fryer?**
Answer- Yes, you can use a baking paper or aluminum foil but

you need to make sure that appropriate space is given so that the steam can pass easily.

8.   **How many items can be cooked at a go in an air fryer?**
Answer- You can easily cook two different items at a go in an air fryer but make sure to use the divider. This will help in proper cooking and less time will be consumed.

9.   **Do we need to preheat the air fryer?**
Answer- No, there is no need to preheat the air fryer. However, pre-heating the air fryer for about 4 minutes can help in significant reduction of the cooking time.

10.   **Does air fryer help in making food crispy and tasty?**
Answer- Yes, the food that you cook in an air fryer is as tasty and crispy as it is with frying. One of the main reasons why air fryer cooks tasty and crispy food is because it helps in keeping the outer layer of the food crisp and the inside gets soft.

Ways to use an air fryer

As the reviews you may have read indicated, there are tons of ways to use an air fryer. Many air fryer foods can be cooked in various ways. Here are some ideas of foods that can be cooked in**multiple ways** with an air fryer:

Once you get accustomed to your fryer, you can also try using air fryer dehydrators and advanced baking with the air fryer baking pans.

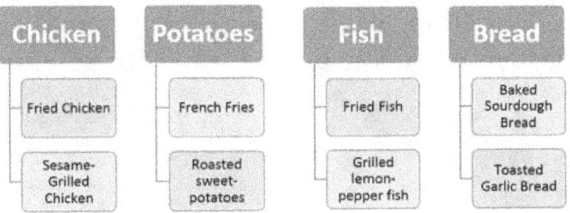

Grill in an air fryer

The best part about grilling with your air fryer is that you do not have to continuously flip your ingredients over for equal heating.

- All you have to do is **shake the pan half way** through the times heating session.
- The hot-air flows around the inside of the appliance, heating up all sides of your food.
- Most air fryers come with either a grill layer or a grill pan that has a handle. This makes it easy for you to insert and remove food from the fryer.
- The surface of the grill can quickly soak up any excess fat that drips from ingredients, leaving you with healthy, grilled to perfection meals.

Bake in an air fryer

Baking in a fryer? That's something you don't hear every day.

With most air fryers, you can use the provided baking pan to make goodies such as muffins, brownies, cupcakes and bread.

Whether you want to make a homemade good or bake pre-heated foods, the air fryer will allow you to do it all. Baking with an air fryer usually takes anywhere from **15 minutes and up to 30 minutes.**

Roast in an air fryer

Too busy to make dinner for your date? Don't worry. With your air fryer, you can roast your meats and veggies for the perfect romantic dinner.

Not only will the fryer produce quality roasted food, but it will also **roast your food 20 percent faster** than your oven.

Imagine that... An air fryer that fries!

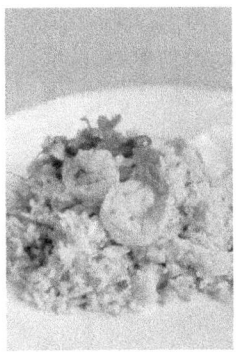

Of course, you can always fry foods in an air fryer. This appliance will give your food the same crisp and mouthwatering taste that an oil fryer would.

However, the biggest factor that differentiates an air fryer from other fryers is that its fried food can be **up to 80 percent less fattening** than food cooked in other fryers.

No oil needed with an air fryer

No oil is needed when making foods with your air fryer.

Even though many people take advantage of using no oil with an air fryer, you can still use it with the fryer. However, you have to mix oil with your ingredients before putting them in the fryer.

- Oil cannot be put inside the fryer pan.
- Adding cooking oil before air-frying, will add an extra crunchy layer to your food.
- Most oils can be used with an air fryer. Some common oils are canola, sunflower, olive and peanut oil.

What foods can I use in an air fryer?

The million dollar question many people ask before purchasing an air fryer is: What kind of foods are for an air fryer?

This question is not surprising because before someone spends their hard earned money on a product, they want to make sure it is useful for them. Luckily, the air fryer can pretty much prepare any food that would normally be cooked in 40 minutes or less on a stovetop, oven or deep fryer.

What kinds of foods are an air fryer suited for?

Meats	
Chicken	Seafood
Pork	Beef

Vegetables	
Peppers	Corn on the Cob
Kale	Zucchini
Asparagus	Cauliflower

Baked Goods	
Cake	Brownies
Muffins	Bread

An air fryer is suited for foods that can be **fried, grilled, roasted and baked.**

- Any foods that require bread crumb or light flour coating, generally for frying, can be used in an air fryer. **Even some veggies** can be used with an air fryer.
- Although both have very different cooking instructions with an air fryer, **home prepared meals and frozen foods** can too be prepared in an air fryer.

What kinds of foods are air fryers not suited for?

Foods that should avoid being prepared in an air fryer are veggies that can be cooked and steamed such as carrots and beans. Also ingredients that will be fried with a batter should be refrained from frying in an air fryer.

What variety of foods can you make with an air fryer?

From chicken to seafood, to corn on the cob and muffins; there are many foods that can be prepared with an air fryer. Below is a list of some of the foods that can be cooked in an air fryer:

Most common ingredient used in air fryers is: Potatoes!

Whether you would like French fries or roasted or grilled potatoes, potatoes are very popular with an air fryer.

You can even make pre-heated frozen fries and potatoes in your fryer. Although frozen foods may take longer to cook in an air fryer, it will not affect the final result of your dish, leaving you with a crispy exterior and soft interior.

Multiple dishes at once

With an air fryer, you can prepare multiple ingredients at the same time. The separator that some of them come with the appliance will enable you to divide the ingredients in the basket or pan and cook both foods at the same time.

However, before cooking multiple foods, you must **ensure that both foods will require the same temperature heating** so they can both cook evenly.

For example, preparing grilled potatoes and shrimp would have different temperature settings because shrimp would not need as high a temperature setting as potatoes.

RECIPES

Blooming Onion

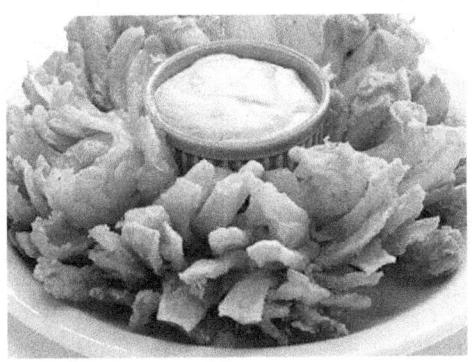

Ingredients

1   Large white onion
0.25 cup Milk, nonfat
2   Large eggs
0.75 cup Panko
1.5 teaspoon Paprika
1 teaspoon Garlic powder
0.5 teaspoon Cajun seasoning
0.5 teaspoon black pepper
1 teaspoon Sea Salt

Directions

1. Mix breadcrumbs with olive oil & Cajun seasoning. In a separate dish, mix salt & pepper. In a bowl, mix milk with egg.
2. Peel onion, cut off top. Place cut side down onto a cutting board.

3. Starting 1½-2 inch from the root, cut downward, all the way to the cutting board. Repeat to make 4 evenly spaced cuts around the onion.

4. Continue slicing between each section until you have made 8 cuts total.

5. Place sliced onion in ice water for at least 2 hours / overnight. Remove from water, pat dry. Open onion so petals are exposed.

6. Beat eggs with 2 Tbsp. milk. Place onion on a tray or in a bowl.

7. Sprinkle onion generously with our mixture. Make sure to get in between all petals. Turn onion upside down to remove excess.

8. Using a ladle, ladle the egg mixture into every crevice. Lift up onion and turn to make sure excess egg drips off.

9. Sprinkle onion very generously with bread crumb mixture. Press into place.

10. Place the blooming onion into the Fry Basket of the Air Fryer. Cover the top with aluminum foil like a tent. Place the Fry Basket into the Air Fryer.

11. Press the M Button to scroll to the Chicken Icon.

12. Press the Power Button & adjust cooking time to 10 minutes at 360 degrees. Leave foil on.

13. When timer is done, check crispness of the onion. Cook 5-10 more minutes to desired crispness.

14. When done, remove carefully and serve with Ranch dressing.

Fried Chicken

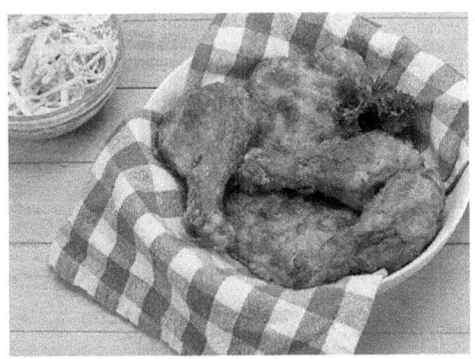

Ingredients

3   Chicken thighs with skin, raw
3   Chicken legs with skin, raw
2 cup Flour, white
1 tablespoon black pepper
1 tablespoon Garlic powder
1 teaspoon onion powder
0.5 teaspoon poultry seasoning
1 teaspoon cumin
1 tablespoon Paprika
1 tablespoon olive oil
1 cup Buttermilk, whole

Directions

1. Soak chicken in buttermilk in the fridge for 2 hours.

2. Add seasonings to the flour. Mix well.

3. Dip chicken into the flour mix, then buttermilk, and back into the flour.

4. Place the chicken into the Fry Basket.

5. Mist chicken with olive oil.

6. Insert Fry Basket into the Power Air Fryer XL.

7. Press the M Button. Scroll to the Chicken Icon.

8. Press the Power Button & adjust cooking time to 20 minutes at 360 degrees.

9. Turn chicken every 5 minutes.

10. Serve when chicken is cooked to desired crispiness.

Hot Wings

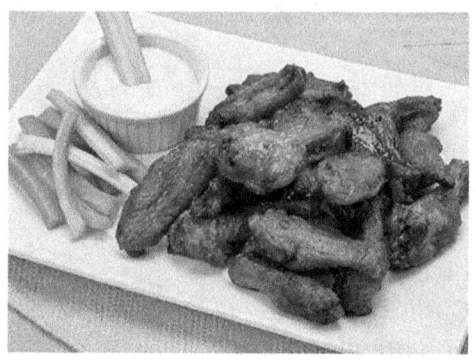

Ingredients

12   chicken wings, drumettes raw
1 cup buffalo sauce

Directions

1.   Place the wings into the Fry Basket and into the Power Air Fryer XL.

2.   Press the M Button. Scroll to the French Fries Icon.

3.   Press the Power Button & adjust cooking time to 25 minutes at 400 degrees.

4.   Half way through the time, ip the wings.

5.   When done remove and toss with the sauce.

6.   Return the wings to the Power Air Fryer XL. Press the M Button. Scroll to the French Fries Icon. 7. Cook for 8 more minutes at 400 degrees.

   8. Toss half way through.

Coconut Shrimp

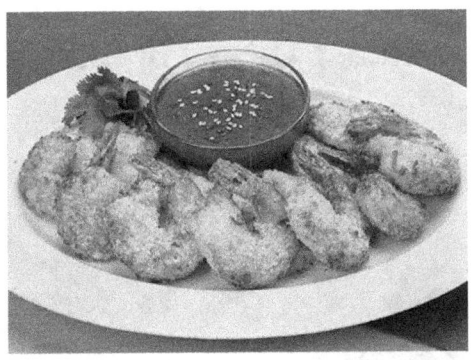

Ingredients
12   large shrimp, raw
1 cup egg white, raw
1 cup coconut, dried, unsweetened
1 tablespoon Cornstarch
1 cup Panko
1 cup Flour, white

Directions
1.   Place the shrimp on paper towels.
2.   Mix the panko and coconut together in a at pan and set aside. Mix the our and cornstarch in a different at pan and set aside.
3.   Place the egg whites in a bowl.
4.   Dip one shrimp at a time into the our mixture, then into the egg whites, and nally into the coconut mixture.

5. Place the coated shrimp into the Fry Basket and repeat until all the shrimp is coated.
6. Place the Fry Basket into the Power Air Fryer XL. Press the M Button. Scroll to the Fish Icon.
7. Press the Power Button & adjust cooking time to 10 minutes at 350 degrees.
8. After 5 minutes, turn if needed.

Roast Turkey Breast

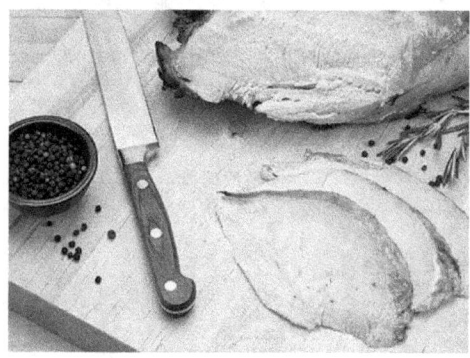

Ingredients

8 pound turkey breast, bone in
2 tablespoon Sea Salt
1 tablespoon black pepper
2 tablespoon olive oil

Directions

1. Season the turkey and rub with olive oil.
2. Place the turkey breast side down in the Fry Basket. Press the M Button.
3. Scroll to the Chicken Icon.
4. Press the Power Button & adjust cooking time to 20 minutes at 360 degrees.

5. When timer is done, carefully turn the breast over.
6. Press the M Button to scroll to the Chicken Icon.
7. Press the Power Button & adjust cooking time to 20 minutes at 360 degrees.
8. Test the turkey with a thermometer for proper doneness (165 degrees).
9. Let rest for 20 minutes before serving.

Cherry Pie

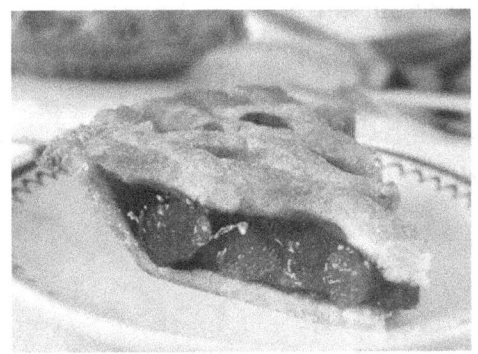

Ingredients
1 21 oz. can cherry pie filling
2 pre-made pie crusts, refrigerated
1 egg yolk
1 tablespoon milk

Directions
1. Press pie crust into the Pie Pan leaving the excess hanging over. With a fork, poke holes on the dough all over.

2. Place the Pie Pan into the Fry Basket and into the Air Fryer.

3. Press the M Button. Scroll to the Bake Icon. Press the Button & adjust cooking time to 5 minutes at 310 degrees.

4. Remove the Fry Basket and carefully remove the Pie Pan. Remove the excess dough hanging over the Pie Pan. Pour the can of cherry filling into the pie crust.

5. Roll the last crust out and cut it into 3/4 inch strips. Place the strips going one way across the top and the opposite way across to make a lattice.

6. Mix the egg and the milk. Brush the pie with the egg wash.

7. Place the Pie Pan into the Fry Basket and back into the Air Fryer.

8. Press the M Button. Scroll to the Bake Icon. Press the Power Button & adjust cooking time to 15 minutes at 310 degrees.

9. When done, let cool and serve with vanilla ice cream or ice cream of your choice.

Mac and Cheese

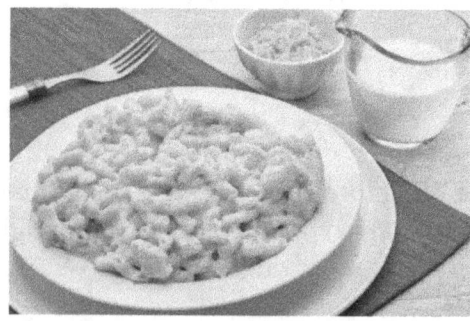

Ingredients
2 cup macaroni, dry
2 cup heavy whipping cream
2 cup cheddar cheese, shredded
1 teaspoon Cornstarch

Directions
1.   Mix the corn starch and then 1 1/2 cups of the cheese together. Place all the ingredients in a bowl and mix.
2.   Pour into the Baking Pan and cover with foil. Place into the Fry Basket and then into the Power Air Fryer XL.
3.   Press the M Button. Scroll to the Bake Icon.
4.   Press the Power Button & adjust cooking time to 15 minutes at 310 degrees.
5.   When the time runs out, open and remove foil. Sprinkle the rest of the cheese on top.
6.   Place the Fry Basket back into the Air Fryer XL.
7.   Press the M Button. Scroll to the Bake Icon.
8.   Press the Power Button & adjust cooking time to 10 minutes at 310 degrees.
9.   Allow to cool before serving.

Country Fried Steak

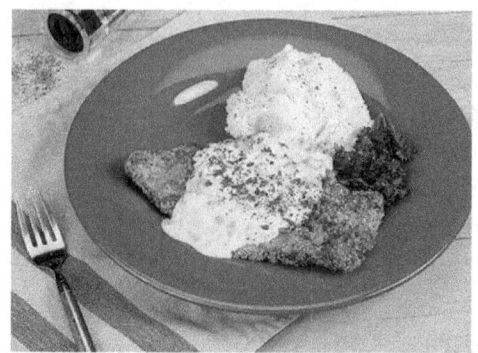

Ingredients

6 ounce sirloin steak-pounded thin
3   eggs, beaten
1 cup flour
1 cup Panko
1 teaspoon onion powder
1 teaspoon Garlic powder
1 teaspoon salt
1 teaspoon pepper
6 ounce ground sausage meat
2 tablespoon flour
2 cup milk
1 teaspoon pepper

Directions

1.   Season the panko with the spices

2.   Dredge the steak in this order. Flour, egg, and seasoned panko

3.   Place the breaded steak into the basket of the Power AirFryer and close. Press the **M** button the Default temperature of 370 F and set the time for 12 minutes. Press the power button

4.   Once the timer has elapsed remove the steak and serve with mash potatoes and sausage gravy.

Sausage Gravy

1. In a pan cook the sausage until well done. Drain fat, reserve 2 tbsp in the pan.

2. Add in the flour to the pan with sausage, mix until all the flour is incorporated

3. Slowly mix in the milk. Stir over a med heat until the milk thickens

4. Season with pepper. Cook for 3 minutes to cook out the flour.

General Tso Chicken

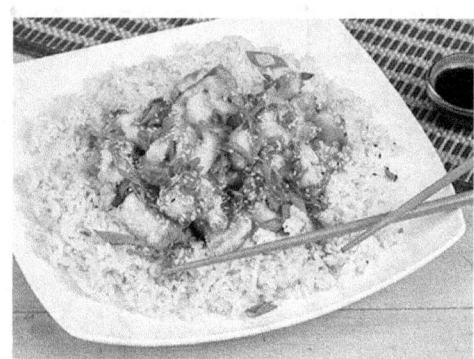

Ingredients

12 ounce Chicken breast, diced
1 cup corn starch
0.25 cup milk
0.5 teaspoon White Pepper
6 ounce General Tso sauce

Directions

1.   Place the chicken in a large bowl. Add in the milk, let sit, drain off milk

2.   Toss the chicken in a bowl with cornstarch, and then shake off excess cornstarch.

3.   Place the breaded chicken into the basket of the AirFryer, close the AirFryer Press the **M** button scroll to the French fry button and set the time for 12 minutes. Press the power button.

4.   Once the timer has elapsed remove the chicken from the AirFryer.

5.   Place the cooked chicken over white rice drizzle sauce over the chicken.

6.   Enjoy.

General Tso Sauce

Wet ingredients

1 tbsp corn starch

3 tbsp rice wine

¼ cups Soy Sauce

3 Tbsp rice vinegar

¼ cup tbsp chicken stock

3 tbsp sugar

Mix these ingredients together

Aromatics

1 tsp Sesame oil

1 tsp ginger minced

1 tsp garlic minced

2 dried whole red chilies

- Add aromatics to a pan warm over med heat. Heat for 2 min
- Add in all the wet ingredients stir until mixture thickens
- Remove from heat cool and reserve for later.

Brie Stuffed Puff Pastry

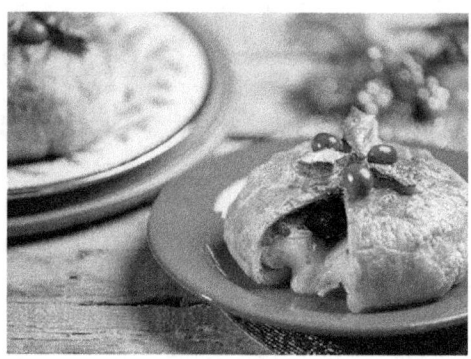

Ingredients

1   sheet puff pastry
0.333333 cup cranberry or lingo berry jam
2   tablespoon Dried Cranberries
2   tablespoon pecans, chopped
1   round 8 oz. Brie
1   egg, for egg wash

Directions

1. On a cutting board sprinkled with a light dusting of flour, roll the puff pastry to remove any imperfections. 2. Use a knife or pizza cutter to remove the four corners of the dough. 3. Spread the jam over the center of the dough, leaving an inch of dough exposed all around. 4. Sprinkle the cranberries and pecans over the jam. Place the round of Brie in the center of the dough. Brush the exposed dough with the egg wash. 5. Fold the dough over the Brie, working in a circle, until the cheese is fully concealed. Use a cookie cutter to cut out decorations for the top of the Brie. 6. Brush the puff pastry with the egg wash. Bake in an Air Fryer at 380 degrees for 7 minutes. Serve warm.

Corned Beef and Cabbage Egg Rolls

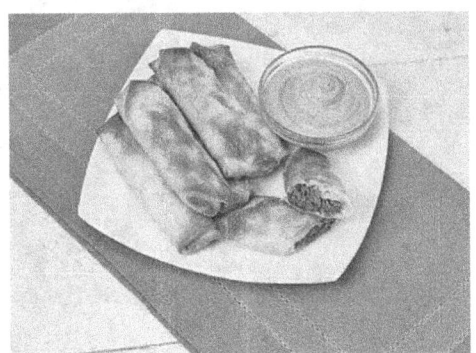

Ingredients

0.75 pound corned beef, shredded
1.5 cup stewed cabbage
12 egg roll wrappers
0 Spicy Mustard

Directions

1. Working with one egg roll wrapper at a time, place the wrapper with one corner of the diamond facing you. 2. Create a small log on the center of the wrapper using about 2 tablespoons worth of shredded corned beef. Top the meat with one tablespoon of the cabbage. Roll the corner closest to you over the filling, and carefully tuck the wrapper to create an airtight seal. 3. Brush the remaining edges of the wrapper with water. Fold in each side of the wrapper, then roll the egg roll up to seal. Repeat until all meat and cabbage are used up. 4. Place the egg rolls in an Air Fryer. Spray the rolls with cooking spray and cook at 400 degrees, for 7 minutes, until golden brown. 5. Serve warm, with spicy mustard.

Clams oreganata

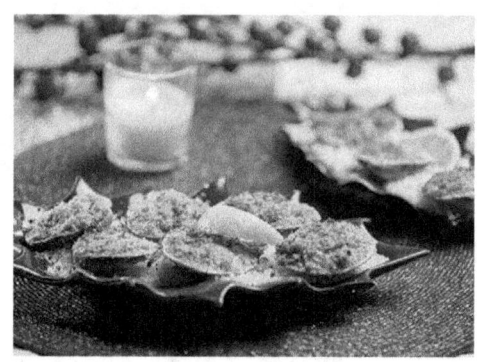

Ingredients

1 cup unseasoned breadcrumbs
0.25 cup Parmesan cheese, grated
0.25 cup parsley, chopped
1 teaspoon dried oregano
3 clove garlic, minced
4 tablespoon butter, melted
2   dozen clams, shucked

Directions

1. In a medium-sized bowl, combine the breadcrumbs, Parmesan, parsley, oregano, garlic, lemon zest and melted butter. Mix to create crumbs. 2. Place a heaping tbsp of the crumb mixture onto the exposed clams. Fill the Copper Chef cake insert with a cup of coarse sea salt. Nestle the clams in the salt and cook at 400 for 3 minutes. Garnish with fresh parsley and lemon wedges.

Roast Pork Loin with Red Potatoes

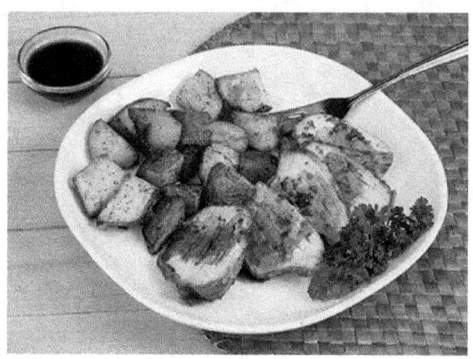

Ingredients

2 pound pork loin
2 red potatoes large dice
1 teaspoon salt
1 teaspoon pepper
0.5 teaspoon Garlic powder
0.5 teaspoon red pepper flakes
1 teaspoon parsley
0 balsamic glaze

Directions

1. Sprinkle the seasonings over the pork loin, and potatoes

2. Place the pork loin, then the potatoes next to the pork in the basket of the AirFryer and close. Press the **M** button scroll to the roast button and set the time for 25 minutes. Press the power button.

3. Once the timer has elapsed remove the pork loin from the AirFryer. Let it rest for a few minutes before slicing

4. Plate the roasted potatoes.

5. Slice the pork. Place 4-5 slices over the potatoes and drizzle the balsamic glaze over the pork.

6. Enjoy.

Fish Taco

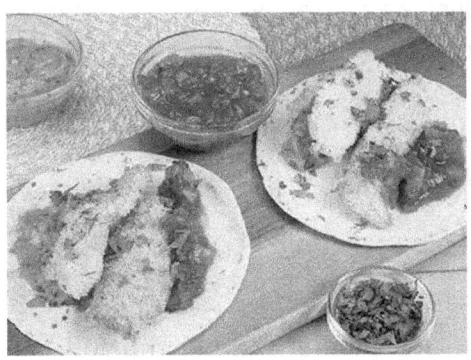

Ingredients

10 ounce cod filet
1 cup Panko
1 teaspoon White Pepper
6 flour tortillas
1 cup tempura batter
1 cup Cole slaw
0.5 cup salsa
0.5 cup guacamole
2 tablespoon cilantro chopped
1 lemon cut into wedges

Directions

1. Cut the Cod filets into long 2 oz pieces, season with salt and pepper.
2. Dip each piece of Cod into the tempura batter, and then dredge in the panko.
3. Place the breaded Cod into the basket of the AirFryer and close. Press the **M** button to scroll to the French Fry button and set the time for 10 minutes. Press the power button
4. Half way through the cooking cycle, turn the fish sticks.

5.   Once the timer has elapsed remove the fish stick from the AirFryer.

6.   Spread guacamole on a tortilla. Place 1 fish stick in the tortilla top with some cole slaw, salsa, and a squeeze of lemon. Top with chopped cilantro. Fold and eat.

Tempura batter

1 cup of flour

1 tablespoon cornstarch

1½ cups of seltzer water cold

Salt

- In a bowl add the flour cornstarch and salt,
- Mix in the cold seltzer.
- Mix all the ingredients together until smooth.

Conclusion

Thank you again for downloading this book!

Part 2

Introduction

In our current changing and fast-paced lifestyles, we are finding less and less time to prepare healthy and nutritious dishes. And with this, there is a machine that could cook food that is not just convenient but also healthy.

And even though Air Fryer is not a significant invention, it undoubtedly changes the life of many people in a better and faster way through cooking.

It also brings up a new cooking lifestyle with health benefits and is not only limited to cooking dishes and entrees but also desserts and snacks such as cakes, cookies, and more!

A Brief Short History Of The Air Fryer

Philips Electronics Company introduced this essential appliance in 2010.

The air fryer is known to be the first kitchen appliance to help people cook food conveniently without getting those unwanted excess fats and oils.

It is invented with the fact that processed foods and fast foods are getting fatter and fatter in which resulting in an unhealthy lifestyle. With this Air Fryer, people cook and prepare meals that are not only nutritious but also low in fat and cholesterol.

From the name, itself, air fryers are known to cook food through the circulation of superheated air. They are usually used to "fry" foods like chips, pastries, chicken, fish, and pretty much anything you feel like frying.

A lot of people are now switching to using an air fryer as it delivers fried food that's perfectly crisped and brown with less fat!

Uses Of The Air Fryer

- Produces low-fat meals. This one's good news for people who are conscious enough with their figure and diet! Since air fryers use hot-air circulation, there's no oil needed to make sure the food is cooked properly. Did you know almost 70% amount of oil is reduced with it? That's a lot.

- Easy to clean. Since the air fryer does not really use oil, cleaning it wouldn't be a fuss for users. Also, its parts are dishwasher safe.

- There's no need to worry about oil spills! So, you won't have to worry about cleaning up a lot of mess and wiping spilled oil everywhere too.
- Air fryers were not only designed to fry! This kitchen wonder can also roast, grill, and bake. How awesome is that?
- The air fryer cools down in a short period of time as it is engineered with a cooling system. Now there's no need for you to wait for a few more extra hours for it to cool down and store it elsewhere.
- No need to worry about having overcooked or undercooked food with the air fryer. Air fryer users are guaranteed to have evenly cooked food as the air around it is heated equally.
- It is safe to use. Air fryers are packed with a variety of safety features. It is also designed with an auto-shutoff feature so there's no need to worry about forgetting it to turn off.
- It heats up in minutes! Fast and efficient – just the perfect terms to describe this kitchen appliance. Newsflash: It cooks food faster than the oven. You can have your own made meal in just a few minutes!

How To Take Care Of Your Air Fryer

Just like any other kitchen appliances, air fryers need some extra attention too! They are easy to clean, yes, but we should do more than that as an owner of one. Proper cleaning and maintenance can help in prolonging the life of an air fryer.

- Use a clean damp cloth when wiping the outside of the air fryer.

- If you prefer not to use a dishwasher, don't forget to wash the pan, tray, and basket with hot water and dishwashing soap.
- Remember to clean the inside of the air fryer with hot water and a clean cloth or sponge.
- Use a brush should there be any food stuck to the heating element above the food basket.
- Do not put the pan, tray, and basket back into the air fryer when they're still wet. Make sure they are completely dry.
- Do not use sharp utensils, or any utensils for that matter to remove any stuck food inside your air fryer as it may damage some components of it.
- Wait for at least thirty minutes to let the air fryer cool down before storing it to safety.
- Inspect its cords.
- Unplug the air fryer from the socket after every use.

How To Use The Air Fyer Even On Diets

Here are some important tips to remember when cooking diet dishes in your Air Fryer:

- Remove the basket from the grease drawer before removing the food. This step is very vital and if you forget this advice, you will surely not make it again after your mistake. If you flip the basket while it is locked to the grease drawer, you will end up dumping the excess oil and fat onto your plate along with the food you just cooked.
- Save the cooking juice and fat. The grease drawer under the cooking basket will collect a lot of flavorful oil and juices from

the food you cooked as well as catch any marinade you pour over your ingredients.

- Flavorful, fatty oils and juices are very useful in the ketogenic diet since you re on a high-fat diet. You can use the drippings as a sauce over your dishes. You can even cook it in a small saucepan for a couple of minutes to make it even more flavorful.
- How to Spend Less Time Cooking
- Cooking food in the air fryer takes less time than cooking them in the oven. But if you want to cook dishes even faster, preheat the appliance to the temperature that you need, set it for 2 to 3 minutes. When the timer beeps, your air fryer is preheated and ready for food.
- Invest in the right accessories. You may need to purchase some valuable accessories for your new favorite cooking appliance once you start air frying. You may already have a couple in your kitchen. You can virtually use any heatproof pan and dish that fits your basket, as long as they do not come in contact with the heating element.
- You can even line the basket with parchment paper or foil for easy cleanup, as long as they are smaller than the air to ensure proper airflow needed for cooking.
- Use a foil sling to put accessory pieces in and getting them out from your fryer. It will definitely be tricky, especially if we have to do it in a hot appliance. You can create an aluminum sling around 2-inch wide and 24-inch long. Place your dish or pan on it, hold the ends of the foil, and lift the container in the basket with ease.
- Tuck or fold the ends of the foil into the basket and return the basket to your air fryer. When the cooking process is done, you can remove the container easily out from the basket by holding the ends of the foil.

After knowing much of the air fryer, why not put it to good use right now?

Here are some easy recipes for you to enjoy using your air fryer! We got you covered from Breakfast to Dinner! Start using your air fryer, and its wonders!

Not Your Ordinary Sweet Potato Fries

Cook and Prep Time: 50 minutes/ Serves: 2 servings

What you need:
For the fries:

- 2 medium sweet potatoes, peeled and cut into 1/4" sticks
- 1 tbsp. extra-virgin olive oil
- 1/2 tsp. garlic powder
- 1/2 tsp. chili powder
- Salt and pepper

For the dip:

- 2 tbsp. mayonnaise
- 2 tbsp. barbecue sauce
- 1 tsp. hot sauce

How to make it:
1. Start by preparing all the ingredients together and your Air Fryer.
2. Then get a large bowl, toss sweet potatoes with oil and spices, and season with salt and pepper.
3. After that, spread an even layer of sweet potato fries in fryer basket in batches then cook at 375° for 8 minutes, flip fries, then cook 8 minutes more.

4. Next, make the dipping sauce by getting a medium bowl, whisk to combine mayonnaise, barbecue sauce, and hot sauce.
5. Serve fries with sauce on the side for dipping.

Enjoy!

Special Baked Potato

Cook and Prep Time: 40 minutes/ Serves: 3 servings

What you need:
- 3 Russet Baking Potatoes
- 1-2 tbsp. olive oil
- 1 tbsp. salt
- 1 tbsp. garlic
- 1 tsp. parsley

How to make it:
1. Start by preparing all the ingredients together and your Air Fryer.
2. Then, wash the potatoes and then create air holes with a fork in the potatoes.
3. Sprinkle the potatoes with the olive oil and seasonings, and then rub the seasoning evenly on the potatoes.
4. After the potatoes are coated, place them into the basket for the Air Fryer and place them into the machine.
5. Air-fry your potatoes at 392 degrees for 35 minutes or until fork-tender.
6. Serve with parsley on top.

Enjoy!

Breakfast Cinnamon Rolls

Cook and Prep Time: 2 <u>hours</u> 30<u> minutes</u>/ Serves: 8<u> servings</u>

What you need:
 For the bread:

- 1 pound bread dough
- ¼ cup butter, melted and cooled
- ¾ cup brown sugar
- 1½ tbsp. ground cinnamon

 For the glaze:

- 4 ounces cream cheese, softened
- 2 tbsp. butter, softened
- 1¼ cups powdered sugar
- ½ tsp. vanilla

How to make it:
1. Start by preparing all the ingredients together and your Air Fryer.
2. <u>For the bread:</u> Start with rolling the dough on a lightly floured surface into a 13-inch by 11-inch rectangle; position the rectangle so the 13-inch side is facing you.
3. After that, brush the melted butter all over the dough, leaving a 1-inch border uncovered along the edge farthest away from you.
4. Next, combine the brown sugar and cinnamon in a small bowl and sprinkle the mixture evenly over the buttered dough, keeping the 1-inch border uncovered.
5. Roll the dough into a log starting with the edge closest to you then roll the dough tightly, making sure to roll evenly and push out any air pockets. Press the dough onto the roll to seal it together after uncovering the edge.
6. And then, cut the log into 8 pieces, slicing slowly with a sawing motion so you don't flatten the dough and turn the slices on their sides and cover with a clean kitchen towel; let

the rolls sit in the warmest part of your kitchen for 2 hours to rise.
7. <u>For the glaze:</u> Start with placing the cream cheese and butter in a microwave-safe bowl and soften the mixture in the microwave for 30 seconds at a time until it is easy to stir.
8. Slowly and carefully add the powdered sugar and stir to combine then add the vanilla extract and whisk until smooth; set aside.
9. Preheat your air fryer to 350ºF.
10. **Next, transfer 4 of the rolls to the air fryer basket and air-fry for 5 minutes.**
11. **Turn the rolls over and air-fry for another 4 minutes then repeat the process with the remaining 4 rolls.**
12. After that, let the rolls cool for a while before glazing.
13. **Spread large scoops of cream cheese glaze on top of the warm cinnamon rolls, allowing some of the glaze to drip down the side of the rolls.**
14. **Serve and enjoy!**

Breakfast Hotdog Sandwich

Cook and Prep Time: 10 <u>minutes</u>/ Serves: 2 <u>servings</u>

-

What you need:
- 2 hotdogs
- 2 hotdog buns
- 2 tablespoons grated cheese

How to make it:
1. Start by preparing all the ingredients together and your Air Fryer and preheat to 390 degrees for about 4 minutes.
2. Then place two hot dogs into the air fryer, cook for about 5 minutes.
3. Remove the hot dog from the air fryer and place the hot dog on a bun, add cheese.

4. Place dressed hot dog into the air fryer, and cook for an additional 2 minutes.
5. You can add mustard and mayo if desired.

Serve and enjoy!

Fish Sandwich

Cook and Prep Time: 15 minutes/ Serves: 4 servings

What you need:
- 4 small cod fillets, skin removed
- salt and pepper
- 2 tbsp. flour
- 40g dried breadcrumbs
- spray oil
- 250g frozen peas
- 1 tbsp. creme fraiche or Greek yogurt
- 10–12 capers
- a squeeze of lemon juice
- 8 small slices of bread or 4 bread rolls

How to make it:
1. Start by preparing all the ingredients together and your Air Fryer then [re-heat the Air Fryer.
2. After that, take each of the cod fillets and season with salt and pepper and lightly dust in the flour. Then roll quickly in the breadcrumbs. Repeat with each cod fillet.
3. Then add a few sprays of oil spray to the bottom of the fryer basket and place the cod fillets on top and cook on the fish setting (200c) for 15 minutes.
4. Meanwhile, cook the peas in boiling water for a couple of minutes on the hob or in the microwave and drain and then add to a blender with the creme fraiche, capers and lemon juice Then taste and blitz until combined.

5. Next, once the fish has cooked, remove it from the Air Fryer and start layering your sandwich with the bread, fish and pea puree.

Serve and enjoy!

Meaty Beef Breakfast Empanada

Cook and Prep Time: 30 minutes/ Serves: 8 servings

What you need:
- 8 empanada discs, in the frozen section, thawed
- 1 cup picadillo
- 1 egg white, whisked
- 1 teaspoon water

How to make it:
1. Start by preparing all the ingredients together and your Air Fryer then preheat the air fryer to 325F for 8 minutes and spray the basket with cooking spray.
2. After that, place 2 tbsp of picadillo in the center of each disc and fold in half and use a fork to seal the edges then repeat with the remaining dough.
3. Next, whisk the egg whites with water, then brush the tops of the empanadas.
4. Lastly, bake 2 or 3 at a time in the air fryer 8 minutes, or until golden and remove from heat and repeat with the remaining empanadas.

Serve and enjoy!

Air-Fried Cereal

Cook and Prep Time: 40 minutes/ Serves: 6 servings

What you need:

- 1/2 cup flaked coconut (unsweetened)
- 1/2 cup shredded coconut (unsweetened)
- 1/2 tablespoon cinnamon ground
- 1/2 teaspoon vanilla extract
- 1/4 cup flaked almonds
- 1/4 cup flaxseeds
- 1/6 cup chia seeds
- 1/6 cup coconut oil melted
- 1/6 cup erythritol
- 1/6 cup pepitas
- 1/6 cup sunflower seed

How to make it:
1. Start by preparing all the ingredients together and your Air Fryer then preheat the fryer to 300F.
2. After that, cut a sheet of parchment paper smaller than the basket area to allow air to flow through then mix all of the ingredients in a bowl till well coated with the liquid ingredients.
3. Then put the parchment in the basket; spread the mixture on the paper cook for 24 to 32 minutes, stirring every 5 minutes to prevent burning.
4. Next, once toasted and golden, remove from the fryer then let completely cool before putting in your airtight container.

Serve and enjoy!

Breakfast Spanish Eggs with Chorizo

Cook and Prep Time: 30 minutes/ Serves: 2 servings

What you need:
- 1 chorizo sausage, diced
- 1 pinch pepper
- 1 pinch salt

- 1 tablespoon olive oil
- 1 teaspoon parsley, finely chopped
- 1 tomato diced
- 1/2 teaspoon paprika
- 1/3 cup roasted peppers, sliced into strips
- 1/4 teaspoon cumin (ground)
- 2 eggs
- 2 ounces manchego cheese, grated

How to make it:
1. Start by preparing all the ingredients together and your Air Fryer.
2. Then put the oil in a frying pan set over medium flame. Add sausage, cumin, and paprika; sauté for 3 to 5 minutes or till the chorizo is fully cooked.
3. Next, add the tomato; cook for 5 minutes or till the tomatoes are very soft. Add the roasted peppers and season with pepper and salt to preference; mix well.
4. Remove the pan from the heat. Preheat the fryer to 370F. Divide the mixture between 2 heatproof dishes. Make a well in the center.
5. Lastly, crack 1 egg into each well. Sprinkle the parsley and cheese on top. Put the dishes in the basket. Cook for 4 to 8 minutes or till the eggs is cooked to desired doneness.

Serve and enjoy!

Easy Air-Fried Granola Bar

Cook and Prep Time: 40 minutes/ Serves: 8 servings

What you need:
- 1/2 tablespoon natvia icing mix
- 1 egg
- 1 tablespoon chia seeds
- 1 teaspoon cinnamon
- 1/2 teaspoon vanilla extract
- 1/4 cup macadamia nuts
- 1/4 cup pecan nuts
- 1/8 cup almonds slivered
- 1/8 cup flaxseeds
- 1/8 cup pepitas
- 1/8 cup shredded unsweetened coconut
- 1/8 cup sunflower seeds
- 1/8 cup warm water

How to make it:
1. Start by preparing all the ingredients together and your Air Fryer then preheat the fryer to 325F.
2. After that, put the chia seeds in a bowl; pour in the warm water and let stand for 5 minutes or till thickened.
3. Blend the macadamia and pecan nuts in your food processor, process till chunked small without turning them to flour.
4. Then mix the chunked nuts, coconut, flaxseeds, pepitas, sunflower seeds, and almonds in a bowl. Add the natvia, cinnamon, vanilla, and egg into the thickened chia seeds and mix the nut mixture with the chia seed mixture.
5. Next, transfer to a tin pan that fits your basket lined with parchment paper. Place the pan in the basket; cook for 16 minutes. Remove the pan from the fryer and slice into 8

portions. Transfer the bars on the basket and cook for 12 minutes or till crisp.
6. Lastly, transfer and let cool completely before transferring to an airtight container.

Serve and enjoy!

Classic Lemon Scone

Cook and Prep Time: 40 minutes/ Serves: 4 servings

What you need:
- 1 egg
- 1 tablespoon coconut flour
- 1 tablespoons erythritol, for sprinkling
- 1/2 tablespoon poppy seeds
- 1/2 tablespoon psyllium husk fiber
- 1/4 lemon, juice & zest
- 1/4 teaspoon baking powder
- 1/8 cup erythritol
- 1/8 teaspoon baking soda
- 2 tablespoons butter
- 3/4 cup almond flour

How to make it:
1. Start by preparing all the ingredients together and your Air Fryer then preheat the fryer to 325F.
2. Then, line a shallow, round baking pan that fits your basket with parchment paper. In a mixing bowl, mix the baking soda, baking powder, psyllium husk, coconut flour, and almond flour and whisk in the poppy seeds till mixed.
3. After that, slice the butter into the flour mixture using a pastry cutter, fork, or your hands till the mixture turns to dough. In a different bowl, whisk the egg and the erythritol till frothy.
4. Next, zest the lemon onto a plate and sprinkle with a bit of erythritol; with a fork, mash the zest and the sweetener and set aside to dry and slice the lemon into quarters and squeeze the juice of a quarter into the egg mixture, carefully to prevent any seeds from getting into – pulp is alright.

5. Then pour the egg mixture into the dough; mix well. Transfer the dough into the prepared pan and form into a dome shape and carefully score the dough into 4 triangles using a knife and place in the basket; cook for 16 minutes.
6. Lastly, remove the pan from the fryer. Slice the triangles and separate each portion. Sprinkle with the sugar-lemon; cook for 8 minutes.

Serve and enjoy!

Air-Fried Egg Casserole Recipe

Cook and Prep Time: 40 minutes/ Serves: 4 servings

What you need:
- 1 cup (150 grams) cherry tomatoes
- 1 tablespoon olive oil
- 2 ounces mozzarella balls, fresh
- 4 eggs
- 6 1/2 grams fresh basil
- Salt and pepper

How to make it:
1. Start by preparing all the ingredients together and your Air Fryer.
2. Then slice the tomatoes into quarters or halves and fry them in a skillet with the olive oil till somewhat softened; set aside to cool.
3. After that, crack the eggs to a mixing bowl and chop the basil; add to the egg. Season with pepper and salt to preference; whisk till well mixed.
4. Next, transfer the mixture to a greased baking dish the fits your basket and spread the tomato on top and distribute the mozzarella balls.
5. Lastly, put the dish in the basket; cook for 20-24 minutes at 325F or till the center of the casserole is completely set.

Serve and enjoy!

Low Carb Cheesy Quiche Pepper Recipe

Cook and Prep Time: 50 minutes/ Serves: 2 servings

What you need:
- 1 bell peppers

- 2 eggs
- 1/4 cup ricotta cheese
- 1/4 cup mozzarella, shredded
- 1/4 cup Parmesan cheese, grated
- 1/2 teaspoon powdered garlic
- 1/8 teaspoon dried parsley
- 1/8 cup baby spinach leaves
- 1 tablespoon Parmesan cheese, for garnishing

How to make it:
1. Start by preparing all the ingredients together and your Air Fryer then preheat the fryer to 350F.
2. Then sliced the peppers from top to bottom into equal halves and remove the seeds.
3. In a food processor, blend the ricotta, mozzarella, parmesan, parsley, and powdered garlic. Divide the cheese mixture between the pepper cups, filling them just below the rim and divide the spinach leaves on top of each and push them under the egg mixture.
4. Next, cover the pepper cups with foil. Put them in the basket; cook for 28 to 36 minutes or till the eggs set.
5. Lastly, remove the foil, sprinkle with the parmesan garnish, and set the fryer to the highest temperature; cook for 2 to 4 minutes or till the tops start to brown.

Serve and enjoy!

Bacon Bagels with Sesame Seeds

Cook and Prep Time: 45 minutes/ Serves: 3 servings

What you need:
   For the Bagels:
- 1 1/2 cups grated mozzarella

- 1 egg
- 1 teaspoon xanthan gum
- 2 tablespoons cream cheese
- 3/4 cup (68 grams) almond flour

   For the Toppings:
- Sesame seeds
- 1 tablespoon butter, melted

   For the Fillings:
- 1 cup arugula leaves
- 2 tablespoons cream cheese
- 2 tablespoons pesto
- 6 slices streaky bacon, grilled

   How to make it:
   1. Start by preparing all the ingredients together and your Air Fryer then preheat the fryer to 370F.
   2. After that get a bowl, mix the xanthan gum and almond flour and add the egg; mix till well incorporated and turns to a doughy ball.
   3. Then, in a pot set over a medium-low flame; gradually melt the mozzarella and cream cheese; remove from heat once melted.
   4. Next, add the melted cheese into the flour mixture; knead till well incorporated. If the dough becomes too tough to work, microwave for 10 to 20 seconds and continue mixing and divide the dough into 3 equal portions.
   5. Then roll each into a log and form into join to form a donut. Place the donuts into a sheet of parchment paper smaller than the basket area to allow air to flow through.
   6. After that, melt the butter and brush the tops of the donuts with it. Sprinkle the seeds on top, pressing to adhere well.
   7. Next, sprinkle with powdered onion and garlic, pressing to adhere, if desired. Place the parchment with the donuts in

the basket; cook for 14 minutes and remove from the fryer and let cool.
8. Lastly, spread the bottom halves with cream cheese, top with pesto spread, couple arugula, bacon, sesame seeds, and top with the top halves.

Serve and enjoy!

Keto Pork Sausage Casserole

Cook and Prep Time: 54 minutes/ Serves: 2 servings

What you need:
- 1 egg
- 1/2 cup cheddar cheese, shredded & divided
- 1/3 pound pork sausage
- 1/3 teaspoon dried, ground sage
- 1/6 cup mayonnaise
- 1/6 cup onion, diced
- 2/3 cups green cabbage, shredded
- 2/3 cups zucchini, diced
- 2/3 teaspoons prepared yellow mustard
- Cayenne pepper

How to make it:
1. Start by preparing all the ingredients together and your Air Fryer then preheat the fryer to 350F.
2. After that, grease a baking dish that fits your basket.
3. Get a pan; cook the sausage in a skillet set over medium flame till almost cooked through then add the zucchini, cabbage, and onion; cook till the veggies are tender and sausage is completely cooked and transfer the mixture to the prepared dish.
4. Next get a mixing bowl, then whisk the egg with the pepper, sage, mustard, and mayonnaise till smooth. Add 1/8 cup of

the cheddar; stir to mix and pour the mixture over the veggie mixture. Spread the rest of the cheese on top.
5. Lastly, put the dish in the basket; cook for 24 minutes or till the cheese is melted and light brown.

Serve and enjoy!

Breakfast Lemon Muffins with Poppy Seeds

Cook and Prep Time: 54 minutes/ Serves: 6 servings

What you need:
- 1 1/2 tablespoons lemon juice
- 1 egg
- 1 lemon (zest only)
- 1 tablespoon poppy seeds
- 1/2 teaspoon vanilla extract
- 1/3 teaspoon baking powder
- 1/6 cup erythritol
- 1/8 cup golden flaxseed meal
- 1/8 cup heavy cream
- 1/8 cup salted butter, melted
- 12-13 drops liquid Stevia
- 3/8 cup almond flour

How to make it:
1. Start by preparing all the ingredients together and your Air Fryer then preheat the fryer to 325F.
2. After that, mix the poppy seeds, erythritol, flaxseed meal, and almond flour in a bowl.
3. Get another bowl, stir the heavy cream, egg, and melted butter till smooth the stir in the flour mixture into the egg mixture; mix till well combined.

4. Next, evenly divide the butter between 6 silicone or tin muffin cups. Put the cups in the basket; cook for 14 to 16 minutes or till the tops are slightly browned then remove from the fryer; let stand for 10 minutes to cool.

Serve and enjoy!

Low Carb Breakfast Sausage and Egg

Cook and Prep Time: 60 minutes/ Serves: 4 servings
What you need:
- 1/2 cup almond flour
- 1/2 pound breakfast sausage
- 1/4 teaspoon powdered garlic
- 1/4 teaspoon powdered onion
- 1/8 cup flaxseed meal
- 1/8 teaspoon sage
- 2 ounces cheddar cheese
- 2 tablespoons butter, melted
- 3 tablespoons maple syrup
- 5 eggs
- Salt and pepper

How to make it:
1. Start by preparing all the ingredients together and your Air Fryer then preheat the fryer to 325F.
2. Put a pan on the stovetop over a medium flame then add the sausage; cook, breaking them up in the process.
3. Get a bowl, measure all of the dry ingredients, including the cheese the add the wet ingredients and 2 tablespoons of maple syrup; mix well.
4. When the sausage is crisped and browned, add the rest of the ingredients.

5. Next, line a 4 1/2-square baking pan or similar that fits your basket and pours the sausage mixture into the pan.
6. After that, drizzle the remaining 1 tablespoon syrup on top of extra maple syrup and put the pan in the basket; cook for 36 to 44 minutes.
7. Lastly, remove from the oven once cooked and let cool. Using the parchment paper, remove and lift the casserole out of the pan then slice.

Serve and enjoy!

Air-Fried Sweet Brownie Muffins

Cook and Prep Time: 32 minutes/ Serves: 6 servings

What you need:
- 1 cup golden flaxseed meal
- 1 egg
- 1 tablespoon cinnamon
- 1 teaspoon vanilla extract
- 1 teaspoon apple cider vinegar
- 1/2 cup pumpkin puree
- 1/2 tablespoon baking powder
- 1/2 teaspoon salt
- 1/4 cup sugar-free caramel syrup
- 1/4 cup cocoa powder
- 1/4 cup slivered almonds
- 2 tablespoons coconut oil

How to make it:
1. Start by preparing all the ingredients together and your Air Fryer then preheat the fryer to 325F.
2. Get a bowl then mix all of the ingredients till well combined and line 6 tin muffin cups with paper liners.

3. After that, spoon around 1/4 cup of the batter into each lined cup and sprinkle the tops with the slivered almonds; gently press to adhere.
4. Lastly, put the cups in the basket; cook for 12 minutes or till the risen and the tops set.

Serve and enjoy!

Hot Egg and Bacon Breakfast

Cook and Prep Time: 45 minutes/ Serves: 6 servings

What you need:
- 1 1/2 ounces cream cheese
- 1/4 teaspoon powdered garlic
- 1/4 teaspoon powdered onion
- 2 jalapeño peppers, seeds removed & chopped
- 2 ounces cheddar cheese
- 4 eggs
- 6 bacon strips
- Salt and pepper

How to make it:
1. Start by preparing all the ingredients together and your Air Fryer.
2. After that, par-cook your bacon in the fryer till semi crisped, yet still pliable then save the collected bacon grease.
3. Using your hand mixer, mix rest of the ingredients, including the bacon grease, till well combined, except for 1/2 jalapeno, cheddar, and bacon.
4. Next, grease 6 tin muffin cups then circle 1 bacon on the sides of each muffin cups.
5. Then divide the egg mixture into the wells; do not overfill. Top with the cheddar cheese and garnish each with jalapeno ring, pressing gently to adhere.

6. Lastly, air fry for 16 to 20 minutes at 350F and remove from the fryer once cooked then let cool slightly.

Serve and enjoy!

Low Carb Avocado Bacon Muffins

Cook and Prep Time: 55 minutes/ Serves: 8 servings

What you need:
- 3 eggs
- 3 bacon slices
- 2 tablespoons butter
- 1/4 cup almond flour
- 1/8 cup flaxseed meal
- 3/4 tablespoons powdered psyllium husk
- 1 avocado
- 2 1/4 ounce Colby jack cheese
- 1 1/2 spring onion
- 1/2 teaspoon garlic, minced
- 1/2 teaspoon dried cilantro
- 1/2 teaspoon dried chives
- 1/8 teaspoon flakes red chili
- 3/4 cup coconut milk
- 3/4 tablespoons lemon juice
- 1 teaspoon baking powder
- Salt and pepper

How to make it:
1. Start by preparing all the ingredients together and your Air Fryer then preheat the fryer to 325F.
2. Get a bowl, mix the lemon juice, coconut milk, spices, psyllium, flax, almond flour, and egg; let sit while you cook the bacon.

3. Get a pan set over the medium-low flame, fry the bacon till crisp; adding the butter in the skillet.
4. After that, grate your cheese and chop your spring onion then add the baking powder, cheese, and spring onion the bowl with the batter.
5. Next, crumble the bacon and add into the batter, along with the grease; mix to combine well.
6. And then slice the avocado into halves; remove the seed and the pit.
7. And while still in the shell, slice the avocado flesh into cubes just stopping short to the skin. Scoop the avocado into the bowl with batter; gently fold it into the batter.
8. Lastly, divide the batter between 8 greased tin or silicone muffin cups. Place the cups in the basket; cook for 19 to 21 minutes.

Serve and enjoy!

Keto Cheddar Chive Ham Cups

Cook and Prep Time: 36 minutes/ Serves: 5 servings

What you need:
- 1 1/2 teaspoons garlic, minced
- 1 cup cheddar cheese, shredded
- 1 tablespoon butter, for greasing the ramekins
- 1/2 cup heavy cream
- 1/2 onion (medium), diced
- 1/2 teaspoon salt
- 1/4 teaspoon black pepper
- 2 tablespoons chives (fresh), chopped
- 3 tablespoons olive oil
- 6 eggs (large)
- 6 ounces ham steak, cooked & cubed

How to make it:

1. Start by preparing all the ingredients together and your Air Fryer then preheat your fryer to 370F.
2. After that, heat the olive oil in a skillet and add the onion and cook till browned then stir in the garlic; sauté till the onion is light brown.
3. Get a bowl then mix all the eggs till well combined and divide the mixture between 6 ramekins. Put the ramekins in the basket; cook for 16 minutes.
4. Lastly, remove from the fryer once cooked. Let cool slightly. Serve and enjoy!

Sweet Cinnamon Donut Muffins

Cook and Prep Time: 60 minutes/ Serves: 6 servings

What you need:
For the Donut muffins:

- 1 egg
- 1 tablespoon powdered psyllium husk
- 1/16 teaspoon ground clove
- 1/16 teaspoon ground ginger
- 1/4 cup erythritol, powdered
- 1/4 cup heavy cream
- 1/4 teaspoon orange extract
- 1/6 cup salted butter
- 1/8 teaspoon allspice
- 1/8 teaspoon liquid Stevia
- 1/8 teaspoon nutmeg
- 3/4 cup almond flour
- 3/4 teaspoons baking powder

For the Coating:

- 1/2 teaspoon cinnamon
- 1/8 cup butter, melted

- 1/8 cup erythritol

How to make it:
1. Start by preparing all the ingredients together and your Air Fryer then preheat the fryer to 325F.
2. Get a pan then set over a medium-low flame; cook the butter till brown, stirring occasionally. Once browned, let the butter cool completely.
3. Then mix all of the dry ingredients till well combined and stir in the butter and all the wet ingredients into a different bowl; combine using your electric mixer.
4. Next, sift in 1/2 of the dry ingredients into the wet ingredients; mix using the electric mixer then add the rest of the flour mixture and repeat the process till the mixture forms the dough.
5. After that, divide the mixture between 6 silicone muffin cups. Put the cups in the basket; cook for 16 to 20 minutes or till the brown on the edges.
6. And then melt the 1/8 butter in a saucepan and mix the sweetener and the cinnamon. Brush the top of the muffins with the butter and sprinkle the sugar mixture on top.

Serve and enjoy!

Sausage and Maple Pancake Cups

Cook and Prep Time: 50 minutes/ Serves: 6 servings

What you need:
- 1 tablespoon powdered psyllium husk
- 1/2 teaspoon baking powder
- 1/2 teaspoon vanilla extract
- 1/8 cup erythritol
- 1/8 teaspoon salt
- 10 drops liquid Stevia
- 2 eggs (large)
- 2 tablespoons coconut milk

- 2 tablespoons maple syrup (Recipe Here)
- 3 ounces ground sausage
- 3/4 cup almond flour

How to make it:
1. Start by preparing all the ingredients together and your Air Fryer then preheat the fryer to 325F.
2. After that, slice the sausage into small chunks; cook in a pan till seared.
3. Then measure the wet ingredients into a bowl; measure the dry ingredients into a different bowl.
4. Next, mix the dry and wet ingredients till combined. Add the sausage; mix to incorporate.
5. Then divide the mixture between 6 muffin cups. Put the cups in the basket; cook for 16 to 20 minutes. Remove from the fryer; let cool for 5 minutes.
6. Lastly, remove from the cups and let cool enough to eat.

Serve and enjoy!

Maple and Peanut Muffins

Cook and Prep Time: 50 minutes/ Serves: 6 servings

What you need:
- 1 egg
- 1 teaspoon maple extract
- 1/2 cup almond flour
- 1/2 teaspoon vanilla extract
- 1/4 cup coconut oil
- 1/4 cup golden flaxseed
- 1/4 teaspoon baking soda
- 1/4 teaspoon apple cider vinegar
- 1/8 cup erythritol
- 1/8 teaspoon liquid Stevia
- 3/8 cup pecan halves

How to make it:
1. Start by preparing all the ingredients together and your Air Fryer then preheat the fryer to 305F.
2. Then chop the pecans in your food processor and transfer 2/3 of the nuts in a mixing bowl; save the 1/3 for later.
3. After that, put all your wet ingredients in another container then put all the dry ingredients in the bowl with pecans; mix well.
4. Mix the wet mixture into the dry mix. Divide the mixture between 6 muffin cups then sprinkle the top with the reserved pecans.
5. Lastly, put the cups in the basket; cook for 20 to 24 minutes.

Serve and enjoy!

Cheesy Sausage Pie Recipe

Cook and Prep Time: 50 minutes/ Serves: 2 servings

What you need:
- 1 1/2 bacon & cheddar chicken sausages
- 1/2 teaspoon rosemary
- 1/4 cup coconut flour
- 1/4 cup coconut oil
- 1/4 teaspoon baking soda
- 1/4 teaspoon cayenne pepper
- 1/8 teaspoon salt
- 2 tablespoons coconut milk
- 2 teaspoons lemon juice
- 3/4 cup cheddar cheese, grated
- 5 egg yolks

How to make it:
1. Start by preparing all the ingredients together and your Air Fryer then preheat the fryer to 325F.

2. Then slice the sausage into small chunks and fry them in a skillet set over medium flame; separate the whites and the yolks of the eggs; save the whites for other dishes.
3. After that, measure all the spiced and dry ingredients into a bowl; mix till well combined and whisk the yolks for 4 to 5 minutes or till creamy then add the coconut milk, coconut oil, and lemon juice; whisk till combined.
4. Next, carefully add the wet ingredients into the dry mix till combined and fold 1/2 cup of the cheddar into the batter.
5. Divide the batter between 2 ramekins, filling each 3/4 full then press the sausage into the batter tops, distributing them evenly.
6. Next, put the ramekins in the basket; cook for 16 to 20 minutes or till the tops are golden. Sprinkle with the remaining cheese.
7. Lastly, set your fryer to the highest temperature and cook for 3 to 4 minutes or till the cheese melted and slightly brown.

Breakfast Cardamom Pumpkin Donut

Cook and Prep Time: 45 minutes/ Serves: 9 servings

What you need:
- 1 egg
- 1 teaspoon powdered psyllium husk
- 1/4 cup coconut flour
- 1/4 cup pumpkin puree
- 1/4 cup ricotta cheese, full fat
- 1/4 teaspoon cardamom
- 1/4 teaspoon pumpkin pie spice
- 1/8 cup butter, salted
- 1/8 cup erythritol

How to make it:
1. Start by preparing all the ingredients together and your Air Fryer.

2. After that, put all the wet ingredients in a bowl; blend with your immersion blender till smooth.
3. Get another bowl then mix all the dry ingredients, except for the erythritol. Slowly mix the dry mix into the wet ingredients.
4. Once the mixture starts to form the dough, add the erythritol/stevia; stir to mix.
5. Next, by 1 1/2 tablespoons, roll the dough into balls using clean hands, making about 9 balls then cut a sheet of parchment paper smaller than the basket area to allow air to flow through.
6. After that, put the balls in the parchment. Air fry for 16 to 20 minutes at 305F, flipping halfway through, or till the outside is light golden brown and slightly crumbly to touch.
7. Meanwhile, mix 1/2 teaspoon pumpkin pie spice with 1/2 to 1 tablespoon erythritol.
8. Lastly, when the donut holes are cooked, remove from the fryer and sprinkle with the erythritol mixture.

Serve and enjoy!

French Toasts with a Twist

Cook and Prep Time: 50 minutes/ Serves: 6 servings

What you need:
- 1 tablespoon coconut oil
- 1 tablespoons erythritol
- 1/2 tablespoon unsalted butter
- 1/2 teaspoon cinnamon
- 1/2 teaspoon vanilla
- 1/4 teaspoon of salt
- 1/8 cup heavy cream
- 1/8 cup almonds, crushed & toasted
- 1/8 cup peanut butter

- 1/8 teaspoon nutmeg
- 2/6 cup almond flour
- 3 eggs
- 5 drops liquid Stevia

How to make it:
1. Start by preparing all the ingredients together and your Air Fryer then preheat the fryer to 325F.
2. After that, grind the toasted almonds in your food processor into small chunks with large pieces still for texture and transfer to a pan set over medium-high flame and toast.
3. Meanwhile, mix the nutmeg, salt, cinnamon, erythritol, and almond flour.
4. Get a microwavable bowl, microwave the peanut butter, butter, and coconut oil for 30 to 40 seconds then add the butter mixture, heavy cream, stevia, vanilla, and eggs into the flour mixture; mix well.
5. Next, divide the batter between 6 muffin cups, making 5 whole and an extra 1/2 muffin and top with the toasted almonds; put the cups in the basket; cook for 16 to 20 minutes.
6. Once cooked, remove from the fryer and let cool for 5 minutes and remove from the muffin cups.
7. Lastly, remove from the molds; let cool for 10 to 15 minutes.
8. Serve with whipped cream.

Enjoy!

Fully Loaded Muffins

Cook and Prep Time: 50 minutes/ Serves: 4 servings

What you need:
- 1 1/2 bars dark chocolate squares, chunked
- 1 egg
- 1 teaspoons vanilla
- 1/4 cup erythritol
- 1/4 cup pumpkin puree
- 1/4 cup salted pistachios
- 1/4 teaspoon baking soda
- 1/4 teaspoon cloves
- 1/4 teaspoon ginger
- 1/4 teaspoon nutmeg
- 1/4 teaspoon apple cider vinegar
- 1/8 cup coconut oil
- 3/4 cup almond flour
- 3/4 teaspoon cinnamon

How to make it:
1. Start by preparing all the ingredients together and your Air Fryer then preheat the fryer to 305F.
2. Get a mixing bowl, mix the spices, baking soda, erythritol, and almond flour till well combined.
3. Then in a separate bowl, mix the vinegar, vanilla, coconut oil, egg, and pumpkin puree till well combined.
4. After that, pour half of the wet ingredients into the dry; mix well and add the remaining and mix well.
5. Next, fold in the pistachio and chocolate chunks into the batter and divide between 4 muffin cups.
6. Lastly, put the cups in the basket; cook for 20 to 24 minutes or till golden brown.

Serve and enjoy!

Crispy and Savory Bacon Frittata Muffins

Cook and Prep Time: 40 minutes/ Serves: 7 servings

What you need:
- 1 cup cheddar cheese
- 1/2 teaspoon ground black pepper
- 1/2 teaspoon cayenne pepper
- 1/2 teaspoon celery salt
- 1/2 teaspoon powdered onion
- 18 bacon slices
- 4 tablespoons heavy cream
- 7 eggs

How to make it:
1. Start by preparing all the ingredients together and your Air Fryer then preheat the fryer to 350F.
2. Then slice the bacon crosswise into halves; mold the slices on the bottom and the sides of 7-8 silicone muffin cups, using 2 half bacon slices for each cup. Put the cups in the fryer; cook for 12 minutes to par-cook.
3. Meanwhile, whisk the spices, cream, and eggs till well mixed, adding your preferred herbs if desired.
4. And then when the bacon cups are par-cooked, place 1 to 2 tablespoons cheddar cheese in the bottom.
5. Next, pour around 1/4 cup of the cheese mixture into each mold, making sure not to let any of it leak out if possible.
6. Lastly, cook for 9 to 12 minutes or till the tops start to brown and remove from the fryer and let cool.

Serve and enjoy!

Low Carb Bacon Frittata

Cook and Prep Time: 45 minutes/ Serves: 4 servings

What you need:
- 1 teaspoon dried parsley
- 1/2 tablespoon butter
- 1/4 cup cheddar cheese
- 1/4 cup half-&-half
- 3 ounces bacon, cooked & chopped
- 4 eggs
- Chopped spring onion
- Minced broccoli
- Spinach, sautéed
- Salt and pepper

How to make it:
1. Start by preparing all the ingredients together and your Air Fryer then preheat the fryer to 350F.
2. After that, grease 4 muffin cups. Mix the half-&-half and the eggs in a bowl till scrambled, leaving some streaks of egg white.
3. Next, fold in the spices, cheese, and bacon and add any ingredients you like.
4. Then divide the mixture between the muffin cups, filling each 3/4 full and put the cups in the basket; cook for 12 to 15 minutes or till the edges are golden and the tops are puffy.
5. Lastly, remove from the fryer; let cool for 1 minute.

Serve and enjoy!

Cheesy Bacon Zucchini Bread

Cook and Prep Time: 65 minutes/ Serves: 6 servings

What you need:
- 1 1/2 ounces almond flour
- 1 ounce coconut flour
- 1 teaspoons baking powder
- 1/2 teaspoon xanthan gum
- 1/4 teaspoon pepper
- 1/4 teaspoon salt
- 2 ounces cheddar cheese, grated
- 2/6 cup butter, melted
- 3 eggs
- 3 ounces bacon, diced
- 3 ounces zucchini, grated then liquid squeezed out

How to make it:
1. Start by preparing all the ingredients together and your Air Fryer then preheat your fryer to 325F
2. Get a bowl, mix the xanthan gum, baking powder, pepper, salt, coconut flour, and almond flour till well combined.
3. Then add the melted butter and eggs; mix well. Fold in 3/4 of the cheddar, bacon, and zucchini and transfer the mixture into a lined 4-1/2 loaf dish or similar that will fit your basket.
4. After that, put the dish in the basket; cook for 28 minutes; top with the remaining cheese.
5. Lastly, cook for 8 to 12 minutes or till the cheese is brown and a skewer is clean when tested in the center then remove from the fryer; let cool for 20 minutes; slice into 6 portions.

Serve and enjoy!

Chicken Breakfast Burrito

Cook and Prep Time: 25 minutes/ Serves: 2 servings

What you need:
- 2 eggs
- 2 whole-wheat tortillas
- 4-ounces cooked chicken breast slices
- ¼ of avocado, peeled, pitted and sliced
- ¼ of red bell pepper, seeded and sliced
- 2 tablespoon salsa
- 2 tablespoons mozzarella cheese, grated
- Salt and pepper to taste

How to make it:
1. Start by preparing all the ingredients together and your Air Fryer then preheat the Air fryer at 390 degrees F.
2. Get a bowl, add the eggs, salt and pepper and beat well.
3. Place the beaten eggs in a small shallow nonstick pan.
4. Arrange the pan into an Airfryer basket and cook for about 5 minutes.
5. Remove egg from the pan then arrange the tortillas onto a smooth surface.
6. In each tortilla, divide the eggs, followed by the chicken slice, avocado, bell pepper, salsa and cheese.
7. Roll up each tortilla tightly like a burrito.
8. Now, set the Airfryer at 355 degrees F.
9. Line an Airfryer tray with a foil paper.
10. **Arrange the burrito into a prepared fryer tray.**
11. **Cook for about 3 minutes or till tortillas become golden brown.**

12. Serve and enjoy!

Lunch Recipes

Cheesy Chicken Taquitos

Cook and Prep Time: 15 minutes/ Serves: 10 servings

What you need:
- 3 cups cooked shredded chicken
- 2 1/2 cups fat-free shredded mozzarella
- 10 small flour tortillas
- 1 lime, juiced
- Cooking spray

How to make it:
1. Start by preparing all the ingredients together and your Air Fryer by preheating to 380 degrees.
2. And then, sprinkle lime juice over pork and gently mix around.
3. After that, microwave 5 tortillas at a time with a damp paper towel over it for 10 seconds, to soften.
4. Next, add 3 oz. of pork and 1/4 cup of cheese to a tortilla then tightly and gently roll up the tortillas.
5. Line each tortilla on a greased foil-lined pan and spray an even coat of cooking spray over tortillas.
6. Air-fry for 10 minutes until tortillas are golden in color while flipping halfway through.

Serve and enjoy!

Beef Tortilla Crunch-Wrap Recipe

Cook and Prep Time: 20 minutes/ Serves: 6 servings

What you need:
- 2 lbs. ground beef

- 2 servings taco seasoning
- 1 1/3 c water
- 6 flour tortillas, 12 inch
- 3 tomatoes
- 12 oz. nacho cheese
- 2 cups lettuce, shredded
- 2 cups Mexican blend cheese
- 2 cups sour cream
- 6 tostadas
- Olive oil

How to make it:
1. Start by preparing all the ingredients together and your Air Fryer and preheat to 400 degrees.
2. Then prepare the ground beef by following the instructions on your taco seasoning.
3. Place 2/3 c of beef, 4 tbsp. of nacho cheese, 1 tostada, 1/3 c sour cream, 1/3 c of lettuce 1/6th of the tomatoes and 1/3 c cheese in the centre of each tortilla then close by flooding the edges up over the center; this should look like a pinwheel.
4. Repeat this process with the remaining wraps.
5. Lay seam side down in your air fryer then spray with oil.
6. Air-fry for 2 minutes or until brown.
7. Carefully flip the wraps and spray again.
8. Cook an additional 2 minutes and repeat with remaining wraps

Serve and enjoy!

Hot Chix

Cook and Prep Time: 20 minutes/ Serves: 4 servings

What you need:
- 1 4-pound chicken
- 2 eggs
- 1 cup buttermilk
- 2 cups all-purpose flour
- 2 tbsp. paprika
- 1 tsp. garlic powder
- 1 tsp. onion powder
- Vegetable oil
- Salt and pepper
- Pickles

For the Hot Sauce:
- 1 tbsp. cayenne pepper
- 1 tsp. salt
- ¼ cup of vegetable oil

How to make it:
1. Start by preparing all the ingredients together and your Air Fryer then pre-heat to 370ºF.
2. After that, cut the chicken to make 8 pieces.
3. **Then in a bowl, whisk the eggs and buttermilk together.**
4. **In a plastic bag or zip-lock, combine the flour, paprika, garlic powder, onion powder, salt and black pepper.**
5. **Next, dip the chicken pieces into the egg-buttermilk mixture, and then toss them in the seasoned flour, coating all sides then repeat this process.**
6. **After that, spray the chicken with vegetable oil and set aside.**
7. **Spray or brush the bottom of the air-fryer basket with a little vegetable oil.**
8. **Air-fry the chicken in batches at 370ºF for 20 minutes, while flipping the pieces halfway through the cooking process; transfer the chicken to a plate and repeat the cooking process onto the next batch.**

9. Then after the second batch, lower the temperature on the air fryer to 340°F and flip the chicken back over and place the first batch of chicken on top of the second batch already in the basket and air-fry for another 7 minutes.
10. For the hot sauce: **Combine the cayenne pepper and salt in a bowl. Heat the vegetable oil in a small saucepan and when it is very hot, add it to the spice mix, whisking until smooth.**
11. **Place the fried chicken on the plate and brush the hot sauce all over the chicken.**
12. **Top with the pickle slices.**
13. **Serve and enjoy!**

Bourbon Bacon Burger

Cook and Prep Time: 35 minutes/ Serves: 2 servings

What you need:
- 1 tbsp. bourbon
- 2 tbsp. brown sugar
- 3 strips maple bacon cut in half
- ¾ POUND ground beef 80% lean
- 1 tbsp. minced onion
- 2 tbsp. BBQ sauce
- Salt and pepper
- 2 slices Colby Jack cheese
- 2 Kaiser Rolls
- Lettuce and tomato

   For the sauce:
- 2 tbsp. BBQ sauce
- 2 tbsp. mayonnaise
- ¼ tsp. ground paprika
- freshly ground black pepper

How to make it:

1. Start by preparing all the ingredients together and your Air Fryer then preheat to 390ºF.
2. Pour a little water into the bottom of the air fryer drawer.
3. Combine the bourbon and brown sugar in a small bowl. Place the bacon strips in the air fryer basket and brush with the brown sugar mixture.
4. Air-fry the bacon at 390ºF for 4 minutes then flip the bacon over, brush with more brown sugar and air-fry at 390ºF for an additional 4 minutes until crispy.
5. Meanwhile, make the burger patties by combing the ground beef, onion, BBQ sauce, salt and pepper in a large bowl then mix together thoroughly with your hands and shape the meat into 2 patties.
6. Transfer the burger patties to the air fryer basket and air-fry the burgers at 370ºF for 20 minutes and then flip the burgers over halfway through the cooking process.
7. Make the sauce while the burgers are cooking by combining the BBQ sauce, mayonnaise, paprika and freshly ground black pepper to taste in a bowl.
8. Next, top each patty with a slice of cheese and air-fry for an additional minute, just to melt the cheese.
9. Spread the sauce on the inside of the Kaiser rolls; place the burgers on the rolls, top with the bourbon bacon, lettuce and tomato.

Serve and enjoy!

All Time Favourite Turkey

Cook and Prep Time: 50 minutes/ Serves: 4 servings

What you need:
- 1 turkey breast, 2 pounds
- 1 tsp. freshly chopped thyme
- 1 tsp. freshly chopped rosemary
- 1 tsp. freshly chopped sage
- 1/4 c. maple syrup

- 2 tbsp. dijon mustard
- 1 tbsp. butter, melted
- Salt and pepper

How to make it:
1. Start by preparing all the ingredients together and your Air Fryer.
2. After preparing, season the turkey breast generously with salt and pepper, then rub all over with fresh herbs.
3. Place in the air fryer and fry at 390º for 30 to 35 minutes or until the internal temperature reaches 160º.
4. Combine the maple syrup, dijon, and melted butter together in a small bowl.
5. Next, remove the turkey from the air fryer and brush mixture all over then return to air fryer and fry at 330º until caramelized for 2 minutes.
6. Lastly, let rest 15 minutes before slicing.

Serve and enjoy!

Crunchy Avocado Fries

Cook and Prep Time: 15 minutes/ Serves: 4 servings

What you need:
- 1 cup breadcrumbs
- 1 tsp. garlic powder
- 1 tsp. paprika
- 1 c. all-purpose flour
- 2 large eggs
- 2 avocados, sliced

How to make it:
1. Start by preparing all the ingredients together and your Air Fryer.

2. Then prepare a bowl and whisk together the breadcrumbs, garlic powder, and paprika. Place flour in another shallow bowl, and in a third shallow bowl beat eggs.
3. Dip avocado slices into flour, then egg, then breadcrumbs mixture until fully coated, one at a time.
4. Next, place in the air fryer and fry at 400° for 10 minutes. Serve and enjoy!

Crispy Fried Pickles

Cook and Prep Time: 55 minutes/ Serves: 3 servings

What you need:
- 2 c. dill pickle slices
- 1 egg, whisked with 1 tbsp water
- 1/2 c. breadcrumbs
- 1/4 c. freshly grated parmesan
- 1 tsp. dried oregano
- 1 tsp. garlic powder

How to make it:
1. Start by preparing all the ingredients together and your Air Fryer.
2. Get a paper towels then pat pickle chips dry.
3. Prepare a medium bowl and stir together breadcrumbs, parmesan, oregano, and garlic powder.
4. Next, dredge pickle chips first in egg and then in the breadcrumb mixture then place in a single layer in air fryer basket and bake at 400° for 10 minutes, do this per batch.
5. Serve with ranch if desired.

Enjoy!

Air-Fried Garlic Parmesan Chicken

Cook and Prep Time: 35 minutes/ Serves: 4 servings

What you need:

- 4 bone-in, skin-on chicken thighs
- 1 cup breadcrumbs (I use Panko)
- 1 tsp. garlic powder
- 1 tsp. Italian seasoning
- 2/3 c. freshly grated Parmesan
- 2 large eggs
- Salt and pepper

How to make it:
1. Start by preparing all the ingredients together and your Air Fryer.
2. Then season chicken with salt and pepper.
3. Get a bowl then whisk together panko, garlic powder, seasoning, and Parmesan.
4. Get a separate bowl then beat the eggs.
5. Next, dip chicken thighs in egg, and then roll in Panko mixture until fully coated.
6. Air-fry at 360º for about 25 minutes or until golden and cooked through.

Serve and enjoy!

Air-Fried Cheesy Tortellini

Cook and Prep Time: 25 minutes/ Serves: 6 servings

What you need:
- 1 package cheese tortellini
- 1 cup breadcrumbs (I use Panko)
- 1/3 c. freshly grated Parmesan
- 1 tsp. dried oregano
- 1/2 tsp. garlic powder
- 1/2 tsp. crushed red pepper flakes
- 1 c. all-purpose flour
- 2 large eggs
- Salt and pepper

How to make it:
1. Start by preparing all the ingredients together and your Air Fryer.
2. Cook the tortellini according to the package instructions. Be sure it is al dente. Then drain.
3. Get a bowl then mix together Panko, Parmesan, oregano, garlic powder, and red pepper flakes and season with salt and pepper.
4. Then get a separate bowl and beat the eggs.
5. After that, get a third bowl then pour the added flour.
6. When all is prepared, coat tortellini in flour, and then dredge in eggs, then in Panko mixture and then continue until all tortellini are coated.
7. Lastly, place in the air fryer and fry at 370° until crispy for 10 minutes.
8. Serve with marinara sauce if desired.

Enjoy!

Crunchy Breaded Pork Chops

Cook and Prep Time: 15 minutes/ Serves: 6 servings

What you need:
- Cooking spray, olive oil
- 6 thick center-cut boneless pork chops, fat trimmed
- 1 large egg, beaten
- 1/2 cup breadcrumbs (I use Panko)
- 1/3 cup crushed cornflakes crumbs
- 2 tbsp. grated parmesan cheese, omit for dairy-free
- 1 1/4 tsp. sweet paprika
- 1/2 tsp. garlic powder
- 1/2 tsp. onion powder
- 1/4 tsp. chili powder

- Salt and pepper

How to make it:
1. Start by preparing all the ingredients together and your Air Fryer then preheat your air fryer to 400F for 12 minutes and lightly spray the basket with oil.
2. Then season pork chops on both sides with 1/2 tsp. salt.
3. After that, combine panko, cornflake crumbs, parmesan cheese, 3/4 tsp. salt, paprika, garlic powder, onion powder, chili powder and black pepper in a large mixing bowl.
4. Next, place the beaten egg in another then dip the pork into the egg, and then the crumb mixture.
5. And when your air fryer is ready, place 3 of the chops into the prepared basket and spritz the top with oil.
6. Lastly, cook 12 minutes turning halfway, spritzing both sides with oil then set aside and repeat with the remaining.

Serve and enjoy!

Air-Fried Tandoori Chicken Recipe

Cook and Prep Time: 45 minutes/ Serves: 4 servings

What you need:
- 1 pound chicken tenders each cut in half
- 1/4 cup Greek yogurt
- 1 tablespoon, minced
- 1 tablespoon **garlic**, minced
- ¼ cup **cilantro** or sub parsley
- .5 – 1 teaspoon **Cayenne**
- 1 teaspoon **Turmeric**
- 1 teaspoon **Garam Masala**
- 1 teaspoon Smoked Paprika
- Salt

For setting:
- 1 tablespoon ghee for basting
- 2 teaspoons lemon juice for finishing
- 2 tablespoons chopped cilantro for garnishing

How to make it:
1. Start by preparing all the ingredients together and your Air Fryer.
2. Then prepare a glass bowl and mix all ingredients except the basting oil, lemon juice and 2 tablespoons of cilantro.
3. After that, set your kitchen timer for 25 minutes and turn on your air fryer to 350F for 5 minutes when the timer goes off.
4. After 30 minutes, open up the air fryer and carefully lay the tandoori chicken in a single layer in the basket of your Air Fryer.
5. Using a silicone brush, baste the chicken with ghee on one side and cook at 350F for 10 minutes.
6. Remove and flip over the chicken, and baste on the other side and cook for another 5 minutes.
7. Get a meat thermometer check to see if the internal temperature has reached 165F and take note of this step. It shouldn't be missed!
8. Set on a plate then add lemon juice and mix, and sprinkle with cilantro.

Serve and enjoy!

Air-Fried Fish Fillets with Lemon

Cook and Prep Time: 17 minutes/ Serves: 4 servings
What you need:
- 3/4 cup bread crumbs (I use Panko)
- 1 30g packet dry ranch-style dressing mix

- 2 1/2 tablespoons vegetable oil
- 2 eggs beaten
- 4 tilapia salmon or other fish fillets
- lemon wedges to garnish

How to make it:

1. Start by preparing all the ingredients together and your Air Fryer then preheat your air fryer to 180 degrees C.
2. Get a bowl then xix the panko and the ranch dressing mix together and add in the oil and keep stirring until the mixture becomes loose and crumbly.
3. After that, dip the fish fillets into the egg, letting the excess drip off.
4. Next, dip the fish fillets into the crumb mixture, making sure to coat them evenly and thoroughly and place them into your air fryer carefully.
5. Lastly, cook for 12-13 minutes, depending on the thickness of the fillets.
6. Serve with the lemon wedges.
7. Enjoy!

Air-Fried Sumptuous Turkey Breasts

Cook and Prep Time: 1 hour / Serves: 10 servings

What you need:
- 4 pound turkey breast, on the bone with skin
- 1 tablespoon olive oil
- 2 teaspoons salt
- 1/2 tablespoon dry turkey or poultry seasoning

How to make it:
1. Start by preparing all the ingredients together and your Air Fryer and preheat your air fryer 350F.
2. Prepare the turkey breast and dub 1/2 tablespoon of oil all over.
3. And then season both sides with salt and turkey seasoning then rub in the remaining half tablespoon of oil over the skin side.
4. Air-fried the turkey breast skin side down for 20 minutes and turn over and cook until the internal temperature is 160F using a meat thermometer about 30 to 40 minutes more depending on the size of your breast.
5. Let it cool and then serve and enjoy!

My Version of Air-Fried Chicken Wings

Cook and Prep Time: 10 minutes / Serves: 4 servings

What you need:
- 1 1/2 pounds chicken wings, flats and drumettes separated

- 1 teaspoon kosher salt
- 1 teaspoon garlic powder
- 1/2 teaspoon cayenne pepper

For coating:

- 1/2 cup hot sauce
- 1 tablespoon unsalted butter, melted

How to make it:
1. Start by preparing all the ingredients together and your Air Fryer.
2. Then lay the wings out in a single layer and pat them dry on both sides with paper towels and sprinkle evenly with the salt, garlic powder, and cayenne.
3. After that, put the wings in the air fryer and turn on to 380°F and cook for 25 minutes, removing the basket and tossing the wings with tongs every 5 minutes.
4. After 25 minutes of cooking, increase the heat to 400°F and cook until the skin is crispy and golden brown for 5 to 8 minutes more.
5. Toss the wings with the hot sauce and melted butter if you like.

Serve and enjoy!

Brussels Sprouts with a Twist

Cook and Prep Time: 25 minutes / Serves: 4 servings

What you need:
- 1 lb. Brussels sprouts, cut in half
- 2 tbsp. honey
- 1 1/2 tbsp. vegetable oil
- 1 tbsp. gochujang
- 1/2 tsp. salt

How to make it:
1. Start by preparing all the ingredients together and your Air Fryer.
2. Get a bowl and combine honey, vegetable oil, gochujang, and salt in a bowl and stir then set aside about 1 tbsp. of the sauce.
3. Stir in the Brussels sprouts into the bowl and stir until all sprouts are fully covered.
4. Next, place your Brussels sprouts in your Air Fryer and cook at 360 degrees F for 15 minutes, shaking the basket halfway through.
5. Once 15 minutes is done, increase the temperature to 390 degrees F and cook for 5 more minutes.
6. After cooking, put into a bowl, cover then stir.

Serve and enjoy!

Air-Fried Healthy Fish Sticks

Cook and Prep Time: 40 minutes / Serves: 2 servings

What you need:
- 1-1/2 pound cod
- 1/2 cup tapioca starch
- 2 eggs
- 1 cup almond flour
- 1-1/2 teaspoon dried dill
- 1-1/2 teaspoon onion powder
- 1/2 teaspoon mustard powder
- 2 tablespoons avocado oil
- avocado oil spray
- salt and pepper

For the sauce:

- 1/3 cup avocado oil mayo
- 1 tablespoon dill relish

- 1 tablespoon chopped fresh or dried herbs (dill, parsley, scallions are great here)
- 2 teaspoons lemon juice
- 1/4 teaspoon salt

How to make it:
1. Start by preparing all the ingredients together and your Air Fryer then preheat to 390ºF.
2. After that, pat fish dry with a paper towel and season with a pinch of salt and pepper; cut into small fish sticks.
3. Get a bowl then place the tapioca starch.
4. Get another bowl then whisk the eggs.
5. Using a large bowl, whisk almond flour, dill, onion powder, salt, pepper and mustard powder.
6. Next, dip the sliced fish into the tapioca, shaking off any excess, then into the egg, then dredge in flour mixture. Repeat the process until all fish is coated.
7. Add then the avocado oil to the basket and then spray the air fryer basket generously with avocado spray, and place as many fish sticks in the basket that will fit with plenty of space in between.
8. Spray fish sticks with additional avocado spray to lightly coat and air-fry for 11 minutes, delicately flipping once at 5 minutes.
9. To make the tartar sauce: Combine all ingredients in a medium bowl then set aside; repeat with remaining fish until they have all been cooked through to reach an internal temperature of 145ºF.

   Serve with the sauce.

   Enjoy!

Air-fried Tasty Chicken Recipe

Cook and Prep Time: 35 <u>minutes</u> / Serves: 4 <u>servings</u>

What you need:
- 1 large egg
- 1 pound boneless, skinless chicken thighs, cut into 1 to 1 1/4-inch chunks
- 1/3 cup plus 2 tsp. corn-starch, divided
- 1/4 teaspoon ground white pepper
- 7 tablespoons lower-sodium chicken broth
- 2 tablespoons lower-sodium soy sauce
- 2 tablespoons ketchup
- 2 teaspoons sugar
- 2 teaspoons unseasoned rice vinegar
- 1 1/2 tablespoons canola oil
- 3 to 4 chiles, chopped and seeds discarded
- 1 tablespoon finely chopped fresh ginger
- 1 tablespoon finely chopped garlic
- 2 tablespoons thinly sliced green onion, divided
- 1 teaspoon toasted sesame oil
- 1/2 teaspoon toasted sesame seeds
- Salt

How to make it:
1. Start by preparing all the ingredients together and your Air Fryer.
2. Then beat the egg in a bowl, stir in the chicken, and coat well.
3. In a separate bowl, combine 1/3 cup corn-starch with salt and pepper.
4. After that, transfer chicken with a fork to corn-starch mixture, and stir with a spatula to coat every piece.
5. Then transfer chicken to air-fryer oven racks leaving a little space between pieces.

6. Next, preheat air-fryer at 400°F for 3 minutes then add the battered chicken and cook for 12 to 16 minutes, giving things a shake midway and let dry 3 to 5 minutes.
   After that, whisk together the remaining 2 teaspoons cornstarch with broth, soy sauce, ketchup, sugar, and rice vinegar.
7. Next, heat up canola oil and chiles in a large skillet over medium heat.
8. Once gently sizzling, add the ginger and garlic; cook until fragrant, about 30 seconds.
9. Get the corn-starch mixture then mix a little and stir into mixture in pan.
10. **Increase the heat to medium-high and when the sauce begins to bubble, add chicken.**
11. **Stir to coat; cook until sauce thickens and nicely clings to chicken, about 1 1/2 minutes and then turn off heat; stir in 1 tablespoon green onion and sesame oil.**
12. **Lastly, transfer to a serving plate, and top with sesame seeds and the remaining 1 tablespoon green onion.**
13. Serve and enjoy!

Chicken with Broccoli Zucchini Plates

Cook and Prep Time: 50 <u>minutes</u> / Serves: 1 <u>serving</u>

What you need:
- 1 1/2 ounces cheddar cheese, shredded
- 1 piece (246 grams) zucchini (large)
- 1 tablespoon butter
- 1 tablespoon sour cream
- 1/2 cup broccoli
- 1/2 stalk green onion
- 3 ounces rotisserie chicken, shredded

- Salt & pepper

How to make it:
1. Start by preparing all the ingredients together and your Air Fryer then preheat your fryer to 370F.
2. Then slice the zucchini lengthwise into halves. Spoon out the seeds and discard.
3. After that, scoop the flesh into a bowl, leaving a 1/2 to a 1-inch shell. Pour 1/2 tablespoon of butter into each boat; season with pepper and salt. Place in the fryer basket; cook for 20 minutes.
4. Meanwhile; shred the chicken and measure 3 ounces and then slice the broccoli florets to small chunks.
5. And then mix the chicken and broccoli with the sour cream and season with pepper and salt to taste.
6. When the zucchini is cooked, divide the chicken mixture between the boats. .
7. Sprinkle then with the cheddar on top; cook for 8 to 12 minutes or till the cheese is melted and browning.
8. Serve garnished with green onion and topped with vegan mayo.

Serve and enjoy!

Ham and Cheese Turnover

Cook and Prep Time: 40 minutes / Serves: 2 serving

What you need:
- 1 1/2 tablespoons coconut flour
- 1 3/4 ounce cheddar cheese
- 1 egg
- 1/2 & 1/8 cups mozzarella cheese, shredded
- 1/2 teaspoon Italian seasoning
- 2 ounces ham
- 2 tablespoons almond flour
- Salt & pepper

How to make it:
1. Start by preparing all the ingredients together and your Air Fryer.
2. Then microwave the mozzarella cheese for a minute and then in 10-second bursts, occasionally stirring, till the cheese is melted.
3. After that, put the coconut flour, almond flour, and seasoning in a bowl.
4. Add then the melted mozzarella and start mixing and then after 1 minute, add the egg and mix to incorporate.
5. Next, prepare 2 sheets of parchment paper smaller than the basket area to allow air to flow through and then transfer the dough between sheets of prepared parchment paper; flatten with your hands or roll into an oblong not larger than the size of the parchment.
6. And then measure a long 4-inch wide space on the center of the dough; alternately layer the cheddar and ham on it in a vertical manner, overlapping the filling as needed and leaving around 1/2-inch on top of the oblong clear.

7. Next, cut diagonal strips towards the edges of the dough and create an equal number of strips on the other side; one strip at a time, pull the dough over the filling to cover.
8. Lastly, preheat the fryer to 370F then put the bottom parchment with the turnover in the basket; cook for 12 to 16 minutes or till the top is golden brown.

Serve and enjoy!

Air-Fried Cheesy Hot Dogs Bacon Wraps

Cook and Prep Time: 5 minutes / Serves: 2 serving

What you need:
- 1 ounce cheddar cheese
- 1/4 teaspoon powdered garlic
- 1/4 teaspoon powdered onion
- 3 hot dogs, beef
- 6 bacon slices
- Salt & pepper

How to make it:
1. Start by preparing all the ingredients together and your Air Fryer then preheat your fryer to 370F.
2. Then slice a long slit in the center of your hotdogs.
3. After that, fill the slits with the cheese and wrap each hotdog with 2 bacon slices; secure the ends with toothpicks.
4. Next, put the wraps in the basket; cook for 28 to 32 minutes.

Serve and enjoy!

Crunchy Tofu and Green Salad

Cook and Prep Time: 30 minutes / Serves: 6 serving

What you need:
- 15 ounces tofu, press for 5 to 6 hours to dry

For the marinade:
- 1 tablespoon sesame oil
- 1 tablespoon soy sauce
- 1 tablespoon vinegar (rice wine)
- 1 tablespoon water
- 1/2 lemon, juice only

- 2 teaspoons garlic, minced

    For the Salad:

- 1 stalk green onion
- 1 tablespoon peanut butter
- 1 tablespoon sambal olek
- 1/2 lime, juice only
- 2 tablespoons cilantro, chopped
- 2 tablespoons soy sauce
- 3 tablespoons coconut oil
- 7 drops liquid stevia
- 9 ounces bok choy

    How to make it:

1. Start by preparing all the ingredients together and your Air Fryer.
2. Then mix all the ingredients for the marinade and slice the tofu into cubes and put in a resealable bag; add the marinade.
3. After that seal and put in the fridge, marinate for a minimum of 30 minutes or overnight.
4. Next, preheat the fryer to 325F and cut a parchment paper smaller than the basket area to allow air to flow through.
5. Then place the parchment in the basket and spread the tofu cubes on it; cook for 28 minutes.
6. Meanwhile, mix all of the ingredients for the salad, except for the bok choy, in a bowl and stir in the spring onion and cilantro.
7. Then cut the bok choy into small slices, like slicing cabbage for coleslaw.
8. Lastly, remove the tofu from the fryer and divide the bok choy between 3 serving plates.
9. Drizzle with the sauce and top with tofu.
10. **Serve and enjoy!**

Low Carb Meatballs with Guacamole

Cook and Prep Time: 5 <u>minutes</u> / Serves: 3 <u>serving</u>

What you need:
For the meatballs:

- 1 pound ground chicken (90%/10%)
- 1/2 bell pepper (medium, red)
- 1/2 lime (medium), juice & zest
- 1/2 teaspoon flakes red pepper
- 1/2 teaspoon powdered garlic
- 1/2 teaspoon salt
- 2 green onions (medium), chopped
- 2 ounces cheddar cheese
- 2 tablespoons almond flour
- 2 tablespoons cilantro, chopped
- 2 tablespoons flaxseed meal

For the guacamole:

- Salt & pepper
- 1/4 teaspoon powdered garlic
- 1/2 lime, juiced
- 1 avocado

How to make it:
1. Start by preparing all the ingredients together and your Air Fryer.
2. Then shred 2 ounces of cheddar in a mixing bowl and set aside.
3. After that, prepare all of the veggies then add the chicken and all the veggies in the bowl with cheese.
4. Next, add all of your ingredients; mix evenly than using a tablespoonful, form the mixture into meatballs.
5. Lastly, when the meatballs are cooked, mash all the guacamole ingredients together till smooth.

Serve the meatballs with the guacamole and enjoy!

Keto Basil and Pepper Pizza

Cook and Prep Time: 40 minutes / Serves: 2 serving

What you need:
- 1 egg, organic
- 1 teaspoon Italian seasoning
- 1/2 cup almond flour
- 2 tablespoons cream cheese
- 2 tablespoons Parmesan cheese (fresh)
- 2 tablespoons psyllium husk
- 6 ounces mozzarella cheese
- Salt and pepper

For the Toppings:
- 1 vine tomato
- 1/4 cup marinara sauce
- 2/3 bell pepper
- 2-3 tablespoons basil, chopped
- 4 ounces cheddar cheese, shredded

How to make it:
1. Start by preparing all the ingredients together and your Air Fryer.
2. Then cut a sheet of parchment paper smaller than the basket area to allow air to flow through.
3. After that, microwave the mozzarella for 40 to 50 seconds until completely melted then add the rest of the ingredients for the base; mix well using clean hands.
4. Next, place the dough on the parchment and flatten to a circle.

5. After then, preheat the fryer to 370F then transfer the parchment with the dough in the basket; cook for 8 minutes.
6. Lastly, top with the toppings and cook for 6 minutes more then remove from the fryer, let cool, and slice into 2 portions.

Serve and enjoy!

Hot and Spicy Bacon Pops

Cook and Prep Time: 40 <u>minutes</u> / Serves: 4 <u>serving</u>

What you need:
- 1/4 teaspoon table blend
- 1/8 cup mozzarella cheese
- 1/8 teaspoon pepper
- 1/8 teaspoon salt
- 2 1/2 ounces cream cheese
- 4 bacon slices
- 4 jalapeno peppers

How to make it:
1. Start by preparing all the ingredients together and your Air Fryer.
2. Then slice the jalapeno lengthwise into halves and scrape out the seeds and guts with a spoon and discard.
3. After that, mix the spices, mozzarella, and cream cheese in a bowl then pack cheese mixture into each pepper halves.
4. Next, put the halves together to make them whole again and wrap each with a bacon slice, starting from the bottom upwards.
5. Lastly, preheat the fryer to 370F and put the poppers in the basket; cook for 16 to 20 minutes. Set the temperature to the highest setting and cook for 1 to 2 minutes.

Serve and enjoy!

Keto Personal Pizza

Cook and Prep Time: 30 minutes / Serves: 4 serving
 What you need:
- 1 vine tomato
- 1/4 cup basil, chopped
- 20 pepperoni slices
- 4 ounces mozzarella cheese
- 4 Portobello mushroom
- 6 tablespoons olive oil
- Salt & pepper

   How to make it:
1. Start by preparing all the ingredients together and your Air Fryer and preheat the fryer to the highest temperature setting.
2. Then scrape the innards and the meat out from the mushrooms till only the shell remains and
3. After that, rub the insides of the shells with 3 tablespoons of olive oil; rubbing it in and season with pepper and salt.
4. Next, create a foil container smaller than the basket area to allow air to flow through and put the shells in the container and place it in the basket; cook for 3 to 4 minutes.
5. After then, flip the mushrooms; rub with the remaining 3 tablespoons, season with pepper and salt, and cook for 4 minutes then slice the tomato thinly into 16 pieces.
6. Lastly, lay tomato slices on each Portobello, top with basil, pepperoni, and mozzarella; cook for 1 to 3 minutes or till the cheese is melted and starts to brown. Remove from the fryer; let cool and serve.

Serve and enjoy!

Special Grilled Ham and Cheese Sandwich

Cook and Prep Time: 35 minutes / Serves: 4 serving

What you need:
- 4 pieces low carb mini buns
- 1 organic egg
- 1 tablespoon coconut oil
- 1 teaspoon coconut flour
- 1/2 teaspoon baking powder
- 1/8 teaspoon salt
- 3/4 tablespoons butter
- 6 tablespoons almond flour

For the sandwich:
- 1 tablespoon butter (salted)
- 2 slices cheddar cheese
- 2 slices muenster cheese
- 3 pieces of mini buns (low-carb)
- 4 slices deli ham

How to make it:
1. Start by preparing all the ingredients together and your Air Fryer then measures the baking powder, salt, and flour in a bowl; mix well.
2. Then microwave the 1 coconut oil and butter in a microwavable bowl for 20 seconds then mix the oil mixture into the flour mixture.
3. After that, whisk the eggs and add to the dough; mix well. Add the coconut flour and mix to thicken then divide the mixture between 4 silicone muffin cups, filling each with 3/4-inch of the batter.
4. Next is preheat the fryer to 325F then put the muffin cups in the basket; cook for 16 minutes or till golden brown.
5. Once done, remove from the fryer; let cool for 10 to 15 minutes before removing from the muffin cups then slice each crosswise into buns.
6. Meanwhile, in a hot pan, cook the deli meat till lightly crisped.

7. Next thing is stacking the cheese in alternating order and slice into quarters then layer ham on the bottom buns and top with the cheese; cover with the top buns.
8. Lastly, in a pan that is set over medium flame; heat the butter. Once the butter is brown, reduce the flame to medium-low then add the sandwiches in the skillet; press down and cook till both sides are crisped.

Serve and enjoy!

Meaty Keto Pizza

Cook and Prep Time: 51 <u>minutes</u> / Serves: 2 <u>serving</u>

What you need:
- 1 cup mozzarella cheese
- 1 organic egg
- 1 teaspoon basil
- 1 teaspoon garlic
- 1 teaspoon pepper
- 1 teaspoon rosemary
- 1 teaspoon thyme
- 1/2 tablespoon oregano
- 1/4 cup Parmesan cheese
- 12-ounces canned, chicken breast
- 3/4 cup low carb tomato sauce

How to make it:
1. Start by preparing all the ingredients together and your Air Fryer and preheat the fryer to 325F.
2. Get a bowl then put the chicken and mash it well.
3. After that, add the egg, parmesan, and all of the spices; mix well.
4. Then transfer the mixture to a tin pan that fits your air fryer basket and press down well using a fork.

5. Next, put the pan in the basket; cook for 12 minutes or till the top is set and the edges are browned.
6. Lastly, spread the sauce on top of the crust and sprinkle with the cheese and air-fry for 12 minutes more.

Serve and enjoy!

Chicken Wings Different Way

Cook and Prep Time: 40 <u>minutes</u> / Serves: 2 <u>serving</u>

What you need:
- 1 tablespoon low sodium soy sauce
- 1 teaspoon garlic, finely chopped
- 1 teaspoon lime juice, fresh
- 1 teaspoon sambal oelek
- 1/2 teaspoon arrowroot starch
- 1/2 teaspoon fresh ginger, finely chopped
- 1/8 teaspoon salt
- 10 chicken drummettes, 1 1/2 pound)
- 2 tablespoons scallions, chopped
- 2 teaspoons honey
- Cooking spray

How to make it:
1. Start by preparing all the ingredients together and your Air Fryer.
2. Then coat the chicken with the cooking spray just make sure the chicken is dry.
3. Place the chicken on their sides in the fryer basket to avoid overcrowding then cook for 25 minutes at 400F; flipping them halfway through cooking.
4. In a small pan, whisk the starch and soy sauce. Whisk in the salt, lime juice, ginger, garlic, sambal, and honey; let come to a simmer over a medium-high flame and cook till the mixture is thick and starts to bubble.

5. Next, transfer the cooked chicken in a bowl then add the sauce; toss to coat

Air-Fried Sweet and Spicy Chicken Drummettes

Cook and Prep Time: 40 minutes / Serves: 2 serving

What you need:
- 1 garlic clove, finely chopped
- 1 tablespoon chives, chopped
- 1 tablespoon toasted sesame oil
- 1 tablespoon low sodium soy sauce
- 1/4 cup rice vinegar
- 10 chicken drummettes
- 2 tablespoons unsalted chicken stock
- 2 tablespoons roasted unsalted peanuts, chopped
- 3 tablespoons honey
- 3/8 teaspoon red pepper, crushed
- Cooking spray

How to make it:
1. Start by preparing all the ingredients together and your Air Fryer.
2. After that, place the chicken in the fryer basket in a single layer then grease well with the cooking spray.
3. Then cook for 30 minutes at 400F, flipping halfway through.
4. Meanwhile, whisk the garlic, red pepper, oil, soy sauce, stock, honey, and vinegar in a pan over a medium-high flame then let come to a simmer and cook for 6 minutes or till thickened, almost like a syrup.
5. Next, transfer crispy drummettes in a bowl.
6. Lastly, add the sauce; toss to coat and serve garnished with the chives and peanuts.

Serve and enjoy!

Keto Spiced BBQ Chicken Wings

Cook and Prep Time: 40 <u>minutes</u> / Serves: 2 <u>serving</u>

What you need:
- 1/8 teaspoon chili powder
- 1/8 cup olive oil
- 1/4 teaspoon powdered garlic
- 1/4 teaspoon pepper
- 1/4 teaspoon ginger powder
- 1/4 teaspoon ground coriander
- 1/2 teaspoon salt
- 1/2 teaspoon paprika
- 1/2 teaspoon erythritol
- 1/2 teaspoon cumin ground
- 1 teaspoon dried thyme
- 1 pound chicken wings

How to make it:
1. Start by preparing all the ingredients together and your Air Fryer then preheat your fryer to 370F.
2. Then put together all the spices, herbs, and the erythritol into a mixing bowl then mix well.
3. After that, add the chicken and toss to coat well with the spice mixture then marinate for 30 minutes then
4. Next, drizzle the wings with the olive oil and place the wings in the basket and cook for 20 to 28 minutes.

Serve with preferred keto dipping sauce.

Dinner Recipes

Air-Fried Italian Meatball

Cook and Prep Time: 35 <u>minutes</u> / Serves: 12 <u>servings</u>

What you need:
- 2 lbs. of ground beef
- 2 large eggs
- 1-1/4 cup bread crumbs
- 1/4 cup chopped fresh parsley
- 1 tsp. dried oregano
- 1/4 cup grated Parmigiano Reggiano
- 1 small clove garlic chopped
- salt and pepper
- 1 tsp. light oil dabbed on a paper towel to coat the air fryer basket

How to make it:
1. Start by preparing all the ingredients together and your Air Fryer.
2. Then place the meat and all the ingredients in a mixing bowl and mix all the ingredients together with your hands until everything is well blended.
3. After that, scoop up a handful of meat and roll in the palm of your hand to your desired size meatball.
4. Next, prepare the Air Fryer according to manufacturer instructions. I lightly coat the basket with avocado oil spread on with a paper towel.
5. And then cook them at 350 degrees for 10-13 minutes until lightly browned then turn them over and cook another 5 minutes; remove to a plate when baked.
6. When the meatballs are ready, place them into the tomato sauce to continue cooking.

7. You can serve with pasta or brown rice.
Enjoy!

Air-Fried Vegan Potatoes

Cook and Prep Time: 35 minutes / Serves: 4 servings

What you need:
- 2 large Potatoes
- 1 to 2 teaspoons olive oil leave out to make oil free
- 1/4 cup unsweetened vegan yogurt
- 1/4 cup unsweetened non-dairy milk
- 2 tablespoons nutritional yeast
- 1 cup chopped spinach or kale
- Salt and pepper

    Topping Ingredients:

- 1/4 cup unsweetened vegan yogurt
- Salt and pepper
- Chopped parsley

-
    How to make it:
1. Start by preparing all the ingredients together and your Air Fryer then rub each potato with oil on all sides.
2. After that you may preheat your air fryer to 390° and when it is already hot,, add the potatoes to your air fryer basket.
3. And then set the cooking time to 30 minutes and when the time is up, turn the potatoes over and cook for 30 more minutes.
4. Next, let the potatoes cool then cut each potato in half lengthwise and carefully scoop out the middle of the potato while leaving enough to create a stable shell of the potato skin and a thin layer of the white part.

5. After that, mash the scooped potato, vegan yogurt, non-dairy milk, nutritional yeast, salt and pepper until smooth and stir in the chopped spinach and fill the potato shells with the mixture.
6. Air-fry on 350 degrees for 5 minutes.
7. Serve with the toppings.

Enjoy!

Honey Sriracha Hot Chicken Wings

Cook and Prep Time: 40 <u>minutes</u> / Serves: 2 <u>servings</u>

-

What you need:
- 1 pound chicken wings, cut into individual drummettes
- 1/4 cup honey
- 2 tablespoons Sriracha sauce
- 1 1/2 tablespoons soy sauce
- 1 tablespoon butter
- juice of 1/2 lime
- cilantro, for garnish

-

How to make it:
1. Start by preparing all the ingredients together and your Air Fryer then preheat your air fryer to 360 degrees F.
2. Then, add the chicken wings to the air fryer basket, and cook for 30 minutes, turning the chicken about every 7 minutes with tongs to make sure the wings are evenly browned.
3. Next, while the wings are cooking, add the sauce ingredients to a small saucepan and bring to a boil for about 3 minutes.
4. After the wings are cooked, toss them in a bowl with the sauce until fully coated.
5. Serve and sprinkle with cilantro.

Enjoy!

Healthy Fully Loaded Quinoa Burgers

Cook and Prep Time: 40 <u>minutes</u> / Serves: 4 <u>servings</u>

What you need:
- 1 cup quinoa
- 1½ cups of water
- 1½ cups rolled oats
- 3 eggs lightly beaten
- ¼ cup minced white onion
- ½ cup crumbled feta cheese
- ¼ cup chopped fresh chives
- Vegetable oil
- 4 whole-wheat hamburger buns
- 4 arugula
- 4 slices tomato sliced
- Salt and pepper

Yogurt Sauce:
- 1 cup cucumber finely diced
- 1 cup Greek yogurt
- 2 tsp. lemon juice
- 1 tbsp. fresh dill chopped
- 1 tbsp. olive oil
- Salt and pepper

How to make it:
1. Start by preparing all the ingredients together and your Air Fryer.
2. To make the quinoa patties: First, rinse the quinoa in cold water in a saucepan, swirling it with your hand until any dry husks rise to the surface.

3. Second, drain the quinoa and then put the pan on the stovetop and turn the heat to medium-high and dry the quinoa on the stovetop, shaking the pan regularly until you see the quinoa moving easily and can hear the seeds moving in the pan.
4. The third step, add the water, salt and pepper and bring the liquid to a boil and then reduce the heat to low or medium-low then cover with a lid, leaving it askew and simmer for 20 minutes.
5. After that, turn the heat off and fluff the quinoa with a fork. If there's any liquid left in the bottom of the pot, place it back on the burner for another 3 minutes then spread the cooked quinoa out on a sheet pan to cool.
6. Next, combine the room temperature quinoa in a large bowl with the oats, eggs, onion, cheese and herbs then season with salt and pepper and mix properly.
7. And then shape the mixture into 4 patties and add a little water or a few more rolled oats to get the mixture to be the right consistency to make patties.
8. Next, spray both sides of the patties generously with oil and transfer them to the air fryer basket in one layer then air-fry each batch at 400ºF for 10 minutes, flipping the burgers over halfway through the cooking time.
9. Meanwhile, make the cucumber yogurt dill sauce by mixing all the ingredients in a bowl.
10. Set your burger on the hamburger buns with arugula, tomato and the cucumber yogurt sauce.
11. Serve and enjoy!

Southern Style Fried Pork Chops

Cook and Prep Time: 25 minutes / Serves: 4 servings

What you need:
- 4 pork chops
- 3 tbsp. buttermilk, fat-free
- 1/4 cup all-purpose flour
- pepper
- salt
- cooking oil spray

How to make it:
1. Start by preparing all the ingredients together and your Air Fryer.
2. Then prepare your pork by washing and patting dry and seasoning with salt and pepper.
3. After seasoning, drizzle the buttermilk over the pork chops then place the pork chops in a Ziploc bag with the flour; shake to fully coat.
4. Next, marinate for 30 minutes to absorb the flavors very well.
5. Then place the pork chops in the air fryer and cook in batches if necessary.
6. Lastly, spray the pork chops with cooking oil then air-fry the pork chops for 15 minutes on 380 degrees and then flip the pork chops over to the other side after 10 minutes.

Serve and enjoy!

Juicy and Tender Chicken Recipe in your Air Fryer

Cook and Prep Time: 17 <u>minutes</u> / Serves: 4 <u>servings</u>

What you need:
- 8 chicken tenders, raw
- canola cooking spray

For the mixture:
- 1 cup breadcrumbs (I use Panko)
- 1 egg

- 2 tablespoons of water

    For the Chicken Seasoning:

- 1/2 tsp. garlic powder
- 1/2 tsp. onion powder
- 1/4 tsp. paprika
- 1 tsp. dried parsley
- Salt and pepper

    How to make it:

1. Start by preparing all the ingredients together and your Air Fryer then preheat your air fryer to 400 degrees F for 5 minutes.
2. After that, get a bowl then whisk the water and egg together.
3. Get another bowl then stir in the panko.
4. In another small bowl, combine all the seasonings for the chicken seasoning.
5. When all is prepared, season the chicken then sprinkle the chicken tenders with the seasoning, turning to coat both sides.
6. After that, dredge the chicken then dip chicken tenders into the egg wash and then press it into the panko and turn to coat both sides.
7. Next, load the Fryer Basket and place the breaded tenders into the fry basket and repeat with remaining tenders.
8. After that, spray a light coat of canola oil or non-fat cooking spray over the panko then press the M button then set to 400 degrees F.
9. Then adjust the cooking time to 12 minutes at 400 degrees. Halfway through cooking, flip the tenders over to brown the other side.

10. ## Serve and enjoy!

My Version of Chicken Nuggets

Cook and Prep Time: 18 minutes / Serves: 4 servings

What you need:
- 1 boneless skinless chicken breast
- 1/4 teaspoon salt
- 1/8 teaspoon black pepper
- 1/2 cup unsalted butter melted
- 1/2 cup breadcrumbs
- 2 tablespoons grated Parmesan

How to make it:
1. Start by preparing all the ingredients together and your Air Fryer then preheat your air fryer to 390 degrees for 4 minutes.
2. Then trim any fat from chicken breast and slice into 1/2 inch thick slices, then each slice into 2 to 3 nuggets.
3. Season chicken pieces with salt and pepper then place melted butter in a small bowl and breadcrumbs with Parmesan in another small bowl.
4. Next, dip each piece of chicken in butter, then breadcrumbs.
5. After that, place in a single layer in the air fryer basket then set the timer to 8 minutes.
6. Lastly, once done air frying, check if the internal temperature of chicken nuggets is at least 165 degrees F then remove nuggets from a basket with tongs and set onto a plate to cool.

Serve and enjoy!

Lemon and Ginger Chicken Recipe

Cook and Prep Time: 1 hour / Serves: 2 servings

What you need:

- 4 Chicken legs with thighs

    For the first row of marinating:

- 1 tsp. Salt
- 2 tsp. Lemon Juice
- 2 tsp. Ginger Garlic Paste
- 1 tsp. Kashmiri Red Chilli Powder

    For the second marinating:

- 2 tbsp. Hung Curd
- 1 tsp. Ginger Garlic Paste
- 1 tsp. Kashmiri Red Chilli Powder
- 1/2 tsp. Black Pepper Powder
- 1/2 tsp. Turmeric Powder
- 1/2 tsp. Cumin Powder
- 1/2 tsp. Garam Masala Powder
- 1 tsp. Coriander Powder
- 2 tbsp. Mustard Oil
- 1 tsp. Lemon Juice
- 2 tbsp. Fresh Cream
- 1 tbsp. Kasuri Methi

    For Toppings:

- 1 tbsp Butter
- 1 tsp Chaat Masala
- Lemon Wedges
- Onion Slices

    How to make it:

1. First, start by preparing all the ingredients together and your Air Fryer.
2. Second, wash the chicken and make 3-4 slits on each piece then mix the ingredients for the first marinade and apply it nicely on the chicken legs.

3. Third, cover the bowl and refrigerate for 5-6 hours. After that, add the ingredients for the second marinade in a bowl and coat the chicken with it.
4. Fourth, cover the bowl and refrigerate for another 4-5 hours then preheat the oven to 180 degrees C.
5. Next, set a dripping tray on the lower half of the oven and set a wire rack above the dripping tray.
6. Then arrange the chicken on the wire rack and grill for 20 minutes and turn the chicken legs and again grill for 15-20 minutes, until they are done.
7. After that, baste the chicken with butter while grilling and remove from oven and brush with butter then sprinkle chaat masala on top.
8. Serve hot with lemon wedges and onion slices.

Enjoy!

Buffalo-Style Cauliflower Recipe

Cook and Prep Time: 20 <u>minutes</u> / Serves: 4 <u>servings</u>

What you need:
- For the Cauliflower:
- 4 cups cauliflower florets
- 1 cup panko breadcrumbs mixed with 1 teaspoon salt

  For the Coating:
- 1/4 cup melted vegan butter
- 1/4 cup vegan Buffalo sauce

  For the dip:
- Vegan mayo or any healthy salad dressing

  How to make it:
1. Start by preparing all the ingredients together and your Air Fryer.

2. Then melt the vegan and then whisk in the buffalo sauce.
3. After that dip each floret in the butter/buffalo mixture, getting most of the floret coated in sauce.
4. Next, hold the floret over the mug until it pretty much stops dripping.
5. After that, dredge the dipped floret in the panko/salt mixture, then place it in the air fryer.
6. Lastly, air-fry at 350F for 17 minutes, shaking a few times, and checking their progress when you shake.
7. Serve with your dipping sauce if you desired.

Enjoy!

Fresh Salmon in Cajun Seasoning

Cook and Prep Time: 15 minutes / Serves: 2 servings

What you need:
- 1 piece of fresh salmon fillet, 200)
- Cajun seasoning
- A light sprinkle of sugar
- a quarter of a lemon Juiced to serve

How to make it:
1. Start by preparing all the ingredients together and your Air Fryer then preheat your air fryer to 180C.
2. Then sprinkle Cajun seasoning all over the salmon just make it is dry and clean and ensure all sides are coated then add a light sprinkling of sugar.
3. Air-fry the salmon fillet about 7 minutes, skin side up on the grill pan.
4. Serve with a squeeze of lemon.

Enjoy!

Healthy Friendly Orange Tangy Tofu

Cook and Prep Time: 40 <u>minutes</u> / Serves: 4 <u>servings</u>

What you need:
- 1 pound extra-firm tofu drained then pressed
- 1 Tablespoon tamari
- 1 Tablespoon corn-starch

For the sauce:
- 1 teaspoon orange zest
- 1/3 cup orange juice
- 1/2 cup water
- 2 teaspoons corn-starch
- 1/4 teaspoon crushed red pepper flakes
- 1 teaspoon fresh ginger minced
- 1 teaspoon fresh garlic minced
- 1 Tablespoon pure maple syrup

How to make it:
1. Start by preparing all the ingredients together and your Air Fryer then cut the tofu in cubes.
2. Then place the tofu cubes in a quart-size plastic storage bag then add the tamari and seal the bag and shake the bag until all the tofu is coated with the tamari.
3. After that, add the tablespoon of corn-starch to the bag and shake again until the tofu is coated.
4. Next, set the tofu aside to marinate for at least 15 minutes.
5. Meanwhile add all the sauce ingredients to a small bowl and mix with a spoon and set aside.
6. Place the tofu in the air fryer in a single layer and cook the tofu at 390 degrees for 10 minutes, shaking it after 5 minutes.
7. When done cooking the tofu, add it all to a pan over medium-high heat.

8. Then stir the sauce and pour it over the tofu and mix the tofu and sauce until the sauce has thickened and the tofu is heated through.

Serve and enjoy!

Seasoned Fresh Fried Catfish

Cook and Prep Time: 1 hour 5 minutes / Serves: 4 servings

What you need:
- 4 catfish fillets
- 1/4 cup seasoned fish fry (I used Louisiana)
- 1 tbsp. olive oil
- 1 tbsp. chopped parsley

How to make it:
1. Start by preparing all the ingredients together and your Air Fryer then preheat Air Fryer to 400 degrees.
2. After that, rinse the catfish and pat dry then pour the fish fry seasoning in a large Ziploc bag.
3. Then add the catfish to the bag, one at a time and Seal the bag and shake; making sure that the entire filet is coated with seasoning.
4. Next, spray olive oil on the top of each filet then place the filet in the Air Fryer basket.
5. After that, close and cook for 10 minutes.
6. Then flip the fish and cook for an additional 10 minutes then flip the fish.
7. Lastly, cook for an additional 2-3 minutes or until desired crispness.
8. Serve and top with parsley.

Enjoy!

Dinner Seasoned Shrimp with Special Sauce

Cook and Prep Time: 30 minutes / Serves: 4 servings

What you need:
- 1 pound raw shrimp peeled and deveined
- 1 egg white about 3 tbsp.
- 1/2 cup all-purpose flour
- 3/4 cup bread crumbs (I use Panko)
- 1 tsp. paprika
- Chicken seasoning
- salt and pepper
- cooking spray

For the sauce:
- 1/3 cup plain, non-fat Greek yogurt
- 2 tbsp. Sriracha
- 1/4 cup sweet chili sauce

How to make it:
1. Start by preparing all the ingredients together and your Air Fryer then preheat your fryer to 400 degrees.
2. After that, season the shrimp with the seasonings then place the flour, egg whites, and bread crumbs in three separate bowls.
3. First, dip the shrimp in the flour, then the egg whites, and the bread crumbs last.
4. Next, spray the shrimp with cooking spray be careful and do not spray directly on the shrimp.
5. Last, add the shrimp to the Air Fryer basket then cook for 4 minutes and open the basket and flip the shrimp to the other side; cook for an additional 4 minutes or until crisp.
6. For the sauce: Combine all of the ingredients in a small bowl then mix thoroughly to combine.
7. Serve the shrimp with the sauce.

Enjoy!

Ground Beef Taco with Fried Egg Rolls

Cook and Prep Time: 40 <u>minutes</u> / Serves: 8 <u>servings</u>

What you need:
- 1 pound 93% lean ground beef
- 16 egg roll wrappers I used Wing Hing brand
- 1/2 onion chopped
- 1 can Cilantro Lime Rotel
- 1/2 can fat-free refried black beans
- 1/2 packet Taco Seasoning I used Trader Joe's
- 1 cup reduced-fat shredded Mexican Cheese
- 1/2 cup whole kernel corn I used frozen
- 1 tbsp olive oil
- 2 garlic cloves chopped
- salt and pepper to taste
- 1 tsp chopped cilantro optional

How to make it:
1. Start by preparing all the ingredients together and your Air Fryer then preheat your fryer to 400 degrees.
2. Then spray a skillet with cooking spray on medium-high heat and stir in the garlic and onions and cook until fragrant.
3. Next, add the ground beef, salt, pepper, and tacos seasoning then cook until browned while breaking the beef into smaller chunks.
4. After that, add the, beans, and corn and stir well to ensure the mixture is combined.
5. And then lay the egg roll wrappers on a flat surface and dip a cooking brush in water.
6. After that, glaze each of the egg roll wrappers with the wet brush along the edges.
7. Next, load the mixture into each of the wrappers.
8. Take note for the egg rolls of this size, double wrap them but if you prefer not to double wrap, you will only need a total of 8 wrappers. Sprinkle each wrapper with cheese.

9. Fold the wrappers diagonally to close and press firmly on the area with the filling, cup it to secure it in place.
10. **And then fold in the left and right sides as triangles and fold the final layer over the top to close.**
11. **Using a cooking brush wet the area and secure it in place and spray each egg roll with olive oil.**
12. **Lastly, load the egg rolls into the pan of the Air Fryer and cook for 8 minutes then flip the egg rolls and cook for an additional 4 minutes.**
13. **Serve with cilantro garnish.**
14. **Enjoy!**

Creamy Mushroom Plate

Cook and Prep Time: 48 minutes / Serves: 2 servings

What you need:
- 1 stalk green onions, chopped
- 1 tablespoon sour cream
- 1/2 cauliflower (large), chopped
- 1/4 cup mushrooms, chopped
- 4 chicken thighs (medium)
- 4 ounces cream cheese

How to make it:
1. Start by preparing all the ingredients together and your Air Fryer then put the chicken in a dish that will fit in your basket.
2. Get a large mixing bowl then mix the green onion, sour cream, and cream cheese.
3. Stir in the mushroom and cauliflower; mix till the veggies are well coated.
4. Next, spread the mixture on top of the thighs and put the dish in the basket; air fry at 325F for 48 minutes.

Serve and enjoy!

Cheesy Air-Fried Eggplant

Cook and Prep Time: 37 minutes / Serves: 4 servings

What you need:
- 1 cup tomato sauce
- 1 egg
- 1 large eggplant, cut into 1/2-inch slices, and make 8 pieces
- 1/2 cup mozzarella cheese, shredded
- 1/2 cup Parmesan cheese, grated
- 1/2 tablespoon Italian seasoning
- 1/4 cup pork rinds, ground
- 4 tablespoons butter, melted
- Salt

How to make it:
1. Start by preparing all the ingredients together and your Air Fryer and preheat your fryer to 360F.
2. After that, put the eggplant rounds in a paper towel-lined sheet pan and sprinkle both sides of the rounds with salt; let sit for 30 minutes to release the moisture and remove some of the bitterness.
3. Next step, mix the Italian seasoning, parmesan, and pork rinds in a plate and set aside.
4. Get a bowl then whisk the eggs.
5. Create a breading station with the egg and pork rinds then melt the butter and grease a dish that will fit your basket with some of the butter.
6. The following step, dip around in the egg, letting excess drip off, and then coat all the sides with the parmesan mixture, shaking excess off and pressing to adhere well.

7. Then put the breaded eggplant in the greased dish and put the dish in the basket; cook for 16 minutes, flip, and cook for 16 minutes or till golden brown.
8. Lastly, top with the marinara sauce and the mozzarella then cook for 5 minutes or till the cheese is melted.

Serve and enjoy!

Spiced Turkey Taco Recipe

Cook and Prep Time: 48 <u>minutes</u> / Serves: 4 <u>servings</u>

What you need:
- 1/2 pound ground turkey
- 3/4 cups cheddar cheese, shredded
- 1/2 cup sour cream
- 1/2 small cauliflower, chopped
- 1/2 teaspoon cumin
- 1/2 teaspoon garlic, minced
- 1/2 teaspoon oregano
- 1/2 teaspoon parsley
- 1/2 teaspoon turmeric
- 1/2 whole jalapeno, chopped
- 1/8 cup chopped red peppers
- 1/8 cup onion, chopped

How to make it:
1. Start by preparing all the ingredients together and your Air Fryer.
2. After that, put the cauliflower and meat in a bowl and add the spices and the herbs; mix till well coated.
3. Next step, stir in the jalapenos, red peppers, and onions.
4. Then mix in 1/2 cup of cheddar and transfer the mixture into a dish that will fit your basket.
5. Lastly, sprinkle the remaining cheese on top then air-fry for 48 minutes at 325F.

6. Serve with scoops of sour cream on top. Enjoy!

Creamy Beef Plate Recipe

Cook and Prep Time: 25 minutes / Serves: 4 servings

What you need:
- 1 cup cheddar cheese, shredded
- 3/4 pounds ground beef (80/20)
- 1/2 & 1/8 cups cottage cheese (small curd)
- 1/2 teaspoon black pepper
- 1/2 teaspoon salt
- 1/4 cup green onions, sliced
- 1/4 cup sour cream
- 7 1/2 ounces enchilada sauce (green)
- 8 ounces cauliflower rice

How to make it:
1. Start by preparing all the ingredients together and your Air Fryer then put the cauliflower in a microwavable bowl; microwave for 4 to 5 minutes or till tender.
2. In a pan set over medium-high heat; cook the beef till browned and add the enchilada sauce and season with pepper and salt.
3. After that, put the green onion, cottage cheese, and sour cream in the bowl with the cauliflower and mix properly till well incorporated.
4. Then transfer the cauliflower mixture into a dish that will fit your basket, spreading to an even layer and spread 1/2 of the meat mixture on top of the cauliflower.
5. Next, sprinkle 1/2 cup of the cheddar on top of the meat and spread the remaining meat on top of the cheese, and sprinkle the rest of the cheddar on top.

6. Lastly, put the dish on the basket and cook for 16 minutes at 325F.

Serve and enjoy!

Creamy Tuna Plate Recipe

Cook and Prep Time: 40 <u>minutes</u> / Serves: 3 <u>servings</u>

What you need:
- 1 1/2 packages shirataki noodles, 339 g
- 1/2 cup heavy whipping cream
- 1/2 of a tuna, 146 grams can
- 1/2 tablespoon butter
- 1/8 cup chopped carrots
- 1/8 cup green onions, chopped
- 1/8 cup mushrooms, chopped
- 1/8 teaspoon xanthan gum
- 6 tablespoons cheddar cheese, shredded
- Salt and pepper

How to make it:
1. Start by preparing all the ingredients together and your Air Fryer.
2. Get a deep pot then set the heat over medium and melt the butter. Add then the carrots, mushrooms, and green onions; sauté for 5 minutes.
3. After that, sprinkle the xanthan gum over the veggies; quickly pour in the cream and stir to mix.
4. Next, the mixture will start to thicken right away; keep the flame on till the mixture starts to bubble then put the noodles in a dish that will fit your basket.
5. Pour in the cream mixture into the noodles and mix in the tuna and cheddar.

6. Lastly, top the casserole with the almond flour if desired, pressing to adhere then put the dish in the basket; cook for 28 minutes at 325F.
7. Serve and enjoy!

Cheesy Pork Rinds Recipe

Cook and Prep Time: 40 minutes / Serves: 3 servings

What you need:
For the sauce:

- 1 – 1 1/2 tablespoons chicken broth
- 1 tablespoon Dijon mustard
- 6 tablespoons mayonnaise

For the Casserole:

- 1 1/2 tablespoons butter, melted
- 1.15 pounds chicken breasts
- 4 slices ham (about 56 grams)
- 4 slices Swiss cheese (about 76 grams)
- Salt & black pepper to preference

For the Topping:

- 1 ounce pork rinds
- 1/4 cup Parmesan cheese, grated
- 1/4 teaspoon powdered garlic
- 1/4 teaspoon salt
- 1/8 cup flaxseed meal

How to make it:
1. Start by preparing all the ingredients together and your Air Fryer and preheat your fryer to 325F.

2. Then blend 1/4 teaspoon salt, garlic, parmesan, flaxseed meal, and pork rinds in your food processor and set aside.
3. After that, take the chicken breasts and slice them lengthwise to create 4 long halves and save 1 breast half.
4. Next, lay the chicken pieces in a dish that will fit your basket; season with pepper and salt.
5. Then again, lay the ham slices on top of the breasts and layer your Swiss over your ham and spread the pork rind mix on top.
6. Drizzle the melted butter over the rind mixture and mix it into the crumbs then put the dish in the basket; cook for 32 to 36 minutes or till the crumb sunk into the melty cheese.
7. Meanwhile, whisk the mustard and the mayonnaise, and then stir in the chicken.
8. Lastly, divide the casserole into 3 portions and topped with the sauce.

Serve and enjoy!

Cheesy Burger Bacon Recipe

Cook and Prep Time: 35 minutes / Serves: 3 servings

What you need:
- 1 1/2 bacon slices
- 1 1/2 pounds ground beef
- 1 egg
- 1 tablespoon low carb ketchup
- 1 tablespoon mayonnaise
- 1/2 tablespoon Dijon mustard
- 1/2 tablespoon powdered psyllium husk
- 1/4 cup almond flour
- 1/4 teaspoon powdered garlic
- 1/4 teaspoon powdered onion
- 132.5 grams cauliflower, riced
- 2 ounces cheddar cheese
- Salt and pepper

How to make it:
1. Start by preparing all the ingredients together and your Air Fryer then preheat your fryer to 325F.
2. After that, put the cauliflower in your food processor and pulse till rice-like and transfer to a bowl.
3. Stir in all the dry ingredients and mix then put the beef and bacon in the food processor; process till slightly pasty and crumbly.
4. Then transfer the meat mixture in a pan and cook over the medium-high flame till brown.
5. Get a large bowl and put the cauliflower, meat mixture, 1 ounce cheddar, and rest of the ingredients.

6. Next, press the mixture into a parchment paper-lined dish that fits your basket and spread the remaining 1 ounce cheese on top.
7. Lastly, put the dish in the basket; cook for 20-24 minutes or till the top is browned then remove from the fryer; let cool for 5 to 10 minutes.

Serve and enjoy!

Air-Fried Nacho Chicken Recipe

Cook and Prep Time: 35 minutes / Serves: 3 servings

What you need:
- 396 grams chicken thighs - skinless, boneless
- 1 1/2 tablespoon parmesan cheese
- 1 tablespoon olive oil
- 3/4 teaspoons chili seasoning
- 1/2 cup green chilies & tomatoes
- 1/2 jalapeno pepper
- 1/2 packet cauliflower
- 1/8 cup sour cream
- 2 ounces cheddar cheese
- 2 ounces cream cheese
- Salt and pepper

How to make it:
1. Start by preparing all the ingredients together and your Air Fryer then preheat your fryer to 350F.
2. After that, chop your chicken and season with pepper and salt then cook with the olive oil in a pan set over medium-high heat till brown.
3. Then stir in the sour cream, cream cheese, and 3/4 of the cheddar; stir till the cheeses are melted and everything is mixed.
4. After that, add the green chilies & tomatoes; mix well then transfer the mixture to a dish that fits your basket.
5. Next, microwave the cauliflower till cooked through and put the cauliflower and rest of the cheddar in a bowl; puree using an immersion blender till the texture is similar to potato mash; season than with pepper and salt.
6. Then again, slice the jalapeno into chunks then spread the cauliflower mash on top of the chicken mixture.

7. Lastly, sprinkle the jalapeno on to, pressing to adhere and put the dish in the basket; cook for 12 to 16 minutes.

Serve and enjoy!

Hot and Spicy Chicken Pops

Cook and Prep Time: 60 <u>minutes</u> / Serves: 3 <u>servings</u>

What you need:
- 1 1/2 jalapenos (medium), de-seed you do not like spicy
- 1 ounce mozzarella cheese, shredded
- 1/8 cup hot sauce (Frank's Red)
- 1/8 cup mayonnaise
- 2 ounces cheddar, shredded
- 3 bacon slices
- 3 chicken thighs (small)
- 6 ounces cream cheese
- Salt & pepper, to preference

How to make it:
1. Start by preparing all the ingredients together and your Air Fryer then preheat your fryer to 370F.
2. After that, remove the bones from the chicken thighs and season the thigh with pepper and salt.
3. Then place the chicken on a trivet set in a foil-lined dish that fits in the basket and cook for 32 minutes, flipping halfway through.
4. After 16 minutes, prepare the filling by chopping the bacon into pieces.
5. Cook in a pan set over medium flame until crisp.
6. Then again, add the jalapeno; sauté till cooked and softened and add the cream cheese, mayo, and hot sauce; stir to mix and season to preference with pepper and salt.

7. Next, transfer the chicken; let the pieces cool slightly. Once cool enough to handle, remove the skins and remove the trivet and foil from the dish.
8. Lastly, lay the chicken in a dish then spread the cheese mixture over them and top with the mozzarella and cheddar; cook at 370 for 10 to 16 minutes.

Serve and enjoy!

Keto Italian Meatballs

Cook and Prep Time: 20 <u>minutes</u> / Serves: 2 <u>servings</u>
What you need:
- 1 1/2 tablespoon flaxseed meal
- 1 1/2 tablespoon tomato paste
- 1 egg
- 1 teaspoon garlic, minced
- 3/4 pound ground beef
- 1/2 teaspoon oregano
- 1/2 teaspoon Worcestershire sauce
- 1/4 cup mozzarella cheese
- 1/4 cup olives, sliced
- 1/4 teaspoon Italian seasoning
- 1/4 teaspoon powdered onion
- Salt and pepper

How to make it:
1. **Start by preparing all the ingredients together and your Air Fryer then preheat your fryer to 370F.**
2. **After that, mix all of the ingredients and form into meatballs then grease the basket with cooking spray.**
3. **Then put the meatballs in the basket in a single layer; cook for 12 to 16 minutes or till the desired doneness is achieved, flipping halfway through.**

Serve and enjoy!

Low Carb Pork Pie Recipe

Cook and Prep Time: 25 <u>minutes</u> / Serves: 2 <u>servings</u>

What you need:
- 1 egg, beaten
- 1/2 pound ground pork
- 1/4 lemon, zest only
- 1/4 teaspoon cardamom
- 1/4 teaspoon ginger
- 1/4 teaspoon ground nutmeg
- 2 tablespoons parmesan cheese, grated
- 2 tart shells, low carb
- Salt and pepper

How to make it:
1. Start by preparing all the ingredients together and your Air Fryer.
2. After that, put the meat and the spices in a pan set over a high flame; once slightly cooked, remove the pan from the heat.
3. Add the lemon zest and egg and transfer the mixture to the prepared tart shells.
4. Cook for 16 to 20 minutes at 325F or till the pork is cooked through then let stand for 5 or 7 minutes to cool.
5. Serve and enjoy!

Beef Chilli Peppers

Cook and Prep Time: 25 <u>minutes</u> / Serves: 2 <u>servings</u>

What you need:
- 1/2 pound ground pork
- 1/2 tablespoon bacon fat
- 1/2 teaspoon chili powder
- 1/2 teaspoon cumin
- 1/2 vine tomato, diced
- 1/4 small onion, minced
- 4 cloves garlic, minced

- 1/8 cup cilantro, packed
- 2 peppers, I use Poblano
- 3 1/2 mushrooms, baby Bella
- Salt and pepper

How to make it:
1. Start by preparing all the ingredients together and your Air Fryer then air fry the poblano peppers using the lowest setting for 8 to 10 minutes, moving and flipping them around every 1 to 2 minutes till all sides are considerably charred.
2. After that, cook the meat in a pan till browned, seasoning with chili, cumin, pepper, and salt then stir in the garlic and onion; cook till softened.
3. Next, add the mushrooms and once the mushrooms absorb the fat in the pan, add the tomato and cilantro; cook for 1 to 2 minutes.
4. Lastly, slice a long slit along one side of each roasted poblano and remove the seeds then spoon the mixture into the poblano; air fry for 6 minutes at 325F.

Serve and enjoy!

Creamy and Cheesy Spinach Pork Roll

Cook and Prep Time: 80 minutes / Serves: 2 servings

What you need:
- 1 1/2 & 1/10 tablespoons olive oil
- 1 1/2 teaspoons garlic, minced
- 1/2 pound pork tenderloin
- 1/8 teaspoon table blend
- 2 1/2 slices prosciutto
- 2 ounces cream cheese
- 3- 3 1/2 cups spinach
- Salt and pepper

How to make it:
1. Start by preparing all the ingredients together and your Air Fryer then preheat your fryer to 400F.
2. After that, butterfly the pork to 1/2-inch thickness and smooth the side using a meat hammer then season with pepper and salt and lightly pound using the spike side of your meat hammer.
3. Next, put the olive oil in a pan and bring it to high heat then stir in the garlic and sauté for around 30 to 60 seconds then add the spinach; sauté till wilted.
4. Then lay the prosciutto slices on the tenderloin, covering the entire surface and spread the spinach mixture on top, leaving the edges clear.
5. Scoop out cream cheese on top of the spinach layer then roll the pork and secure using toothpicks or tie with kitchen twine then season the outside of the roll with the table blend and garlic.
6. Lastly, put the roll on the basket; cook for 16 minutes then reduce the temperature to 305F and cook for 48 to 60 minutes or till the internal temperature reaches 145F.

Serve and enjoy!

Keto Meaty Bacon Wraps

Cook and Prep Time: 60 minutes / Serves: 2 servings

What you need:
- 1 piece 2 pounds pork tenderloins
- 1 tablespoon Dijon mustard
- 1 tablespoon maple syrup, sugar-free
- 1/2 tablespoon soy sauce
- 1/2 teaspoon garlic, minced

- 1/2 teaspoon liquid smoke
- 1/2 teaspoon dried rosemary
- 1/8 teaspoon black pepper
- 1/8 teaspoon cayenne
- 1/8 teaspoon dried sage
- 5 bacon slices

How to make it:
1. Start by preparing all the ingredients together and your Air Fryer then preheat the fryer to 325F.
2. After that, mix all of the wet ingredients to create the marinade then put the pork and dry ingredients in a zip-lock bag and add the marinade.
3. Lock the zip-lock then shake and turn to coat the tenderloin well; refrigerate for 3 to 5 hours.
4. Next, remove the pork from the marinade then wrap with the bacon and put in the fryer; cook for 48 minutes.
5. Then reduce the temperature to the highest setting and cook for 4 to 8 minutes.
6. Lastly, transfer, cover with foil, let rest for 10 to 15 minutes before slicing.

Serve and enjoy!

Keto Baked Ham and Cheese

Cook and Prep Time: 55 <u>minutes</u> / Serves: 3 <u>servings</u>

What you need:
- 1 1/4 cups cheddar cheese, shredded
- 1 cup ham, cooked & chopped
- 3/4 cup heavy cream
- 1/2 cup mozzarella, cubed
- 1/4 cup sour cream
- 1/4 teaspoon black pepper

- 1/4 teaspoon powdered garlic
- 12-ounce frozen cauliflower, chopped

How to make it:
1. Start by preparing all the ingredients together and your Air Fryer then preheat the fryer to 350F and grease a dish that fits your basket.
2. Then put the cauliflower in a pot with water enough to cover the cauliflower.
3. After that, heat on the stovetop and let come to a boil; cook for 8 to 10 minutes or till softened then drain in a colander and return the cauliflower in the pot.
4. Next, puree the cauliflower using your food processor or masher till desired consistency is achieved.
5. Then spread the cauliflower in the bottom of the dish and spread the ham on the cauliflower layer.
6. Get a pan then mix the seasonings, cream, sour cream, and cheddar over medium flame till the cheese is melted slightly.
7. Next, evenly pour on top of the layered ingredients in the dish and sprinkle with the mozzarella on top.
8. Lastly, put the dish in the basket and cook for 32 to 36 minutes or till the top browns.

Serve and enjoy!

Keto Bacon Cheese Bomb

Cook and Prep Time: 55 minutes / Serves: 3 servings

What you need:
- 1 1/4 cups cheddar cheese, shredded
- 1 tablespoon chipotle seasoning
- 1 teaspoons table seasoning
- 16 bacon slices
- 2 1/2 cups spinach

How to make it:
1. Start by preparing all the ingredients together and your Air Fryer then preheat the fryer to 325F.
2. Next, weave the bacon by 10 horizontal pieces and 8 pieces vertical.
3. Once done, season the bacon with your seasoning mix then leaving 1/2-inch of the edges clear and spread the cheese over the bacon weave.
4. After that, spread the spinach on top of the cheeses, pressing down to compress a bit to help you roll it up.
5. Then roll the weave, ensuring that it stays tight and only a bit of filling falls through; some cheese may fall out in the process then season the outside of the weave.
6. Next, place the roll carefully in the basket; cook for 48 to 56 minutes without flipping the roll – the top bacon will be very crisp once done.
7. Lastly, transfer and let cool for 10 to 15 minutes before removing from the before moving and slicing.

Serve and enjoy!

Bread and Brie Beef

Cook and Prep Time: 15 minutes / Serves: 2 servings

What you need:
- 1 cheddar cheese slice
- 1 teaspoon salt
- 1 teaspoon Worcestershire
- 1 wedge (1 1/2-ounce) brie
- 1/2 pound ground chuck
- 1/2 teaspoon table blend
- 1/4 teaspoon ground black pepper

- 1/4 teaspoon powdered garlic
- 2 slices low carb focaccia bread

How to make it:
1. Start by preparing all the ingredients together and your Air Fryer then preheat your fryer to 400F.
2. After that, mix the ground beef with the spices. Reserve around 1/4 cup of the meat mixture to serve as the topping. Form the remaining into a patty. With your knuckle, push a well in the center.
3. And then add the sliced brie in the well and cover the cheese with the reserved meat mixture, pressing to seal the cheese inside.
4. Next, put the patty in the basket; cook for 9 minutes for rare, 10 minutes for medium-rare, 11 minutes for medium, 12 minutes for medium-well, and 13 minutes or more for well done.

Serve and enjoy!

Beefy Bacon Stuffed Bell Peppers

Cook and Prep Time: 25 <u>minutes</u> / Serves: 2 <u>servings</u>

What you need:
- 1 1/2 tablespoons olive oil
- 1 tablespoons ketchup
- 1 teaspoons oregano
- 3/4 pounds ground beef
- 3/4 teaspoons Worcestershire
- 1/2 tablespoon garlic, minced
- 1/2 tablespoon soy sauce
- 1/2 teaspoon hot sauce
- 1/2 teaspoon liquid smoke
- 1/4 teaspoon ground black pepper

- 2 bell medium peppers
- 2 slices thick-cut bacon

How to make it:
1. Start by preparing all the ingredients together and your Air Fryer then preheat the fryer to 325F.
2. Then put the beef and all of the spices in a zip-lock bag; toss, shake, squeeze to mix well and refrigerate for 3 hours.
3. After that, set a pot of salted water on the stovetop and turn on the flame. Meanwhile, remove the cores from the peppers. Once the water is boiling, add the peppers, boil for 3 minutes and remove from the pot to dry.
4. Next, cook your bacon in the fryer till just done and chop then mix in with the beef after marinating is done. Stuff the bell peppers with the meat mixture.
5. Lastly. put the bell peppers in the basket; cook for 40 minutes or till the meat filling is medium hot then top with the cheese and reduce the fryer temperature to the highest setting; cook the bell peppers till the top is charred.

Serve and enjoy!

Mozzarella Bacon Keto Meatballs

Cook and Prep Time: 30 minutes / Serves: 12 servings

What you need:
- 1 egg
- 1 teaspoon garlic, minced
- 3/4 pounds ground beef
- 1/2 cup mozzarella cheese
- 1/2 teaspoon pepper
- 1/4 teaspoon powdered onion
- 1/4 teaspoon salt
- 1/6 cup pork rinds, crushed

- 2 bacon slices
- 6 tablespoons pesto sauce

How to make it:
1. Start by preparing all the ingredients together and your Air Fryer then preheat the fryer to 325F.
2. After that, slice the bacon into small cubes then mix the beef with the bacon, egg, cheese, spices, and pork rinds till well incorporated.
3. Form the mixture into 10 balls and put the meatballs in the basket; cook for 32 to 36 minutes or till the bacon pieces are cooked.
4. Lastly, serve with 1/2 tablespoons of pesto topped on each meatball.

Enjoy!

Cheesy Chorizo Keto Meatballs

Cook and Prep Time: 50 minutes / Serves: 12 servings

What you need:
- 1 egg
- 1/2 cup (56.5 grams) cheddar cheese
- 1/2 cup tomato sauce
- 1/2 teaspoon chili powder
- 1/2 teaspoon cumin
- 1/2 teaspoon salt
- 1/4 & 1/2 link (45 grams) chorizo sausages
- 1/4 & 1/2 pounds ground beef
- 6 tablespoons pork rinds, crushed

How to make it:
1. Start by preparing all the ingredients together and your Air Fryer then preheat the fryer to 325F.

2. After that, break the chorizo into small pieces and mix the beef, sausage, egg, cheese, spices, and pork rind till well incorporated.
3. Then form the mixture into 12 balls and place the meatballs in the basket; cook for 24 to 28 minutes or till cooked through.
4. Lastly, spoon tomato sauce over each serving.

Serve and enjoy!

Pepper and Sausage Italian Meatballs Recipe

Cook and Prep Time: 50 <u>minutes</u> / Serves: 11 <u>servings</u>

What you need:
- 1 1/2 links (169.5 grams) hot Italian sausages
- 1 1/2 pounds ground beef
- 1 cup alfredo sauce
- 1 teaspoon Italian seasoning
- 1 teaspoon oregano
- 1 teaspoon salt
- 1/3 cup pork rinds, crushed
- 2 eggs
- 5 pepper jack cheese slices

How to make it:
1. Start by preparing all the ingredients together and your Air Fryer then preheat your oven to 325F.
2. After that, break the sausage into small pieces then mix the beef, sausage, egg, spices, and pork rinds till well incorporated.
3. Then divide the meat mixture into 11 portions and form into a ball and push in the middle to form a well.
4. Next, divide the pepper jack into 11 portions and place the cheese in the well and seal the cheese inside the ball.

5. Lastly, put the meatballs in the basket; cook for 28 to 36 minutes then spoon Alfredo sauce over each serving of meatballs.

Serve and enjoy!

Baked Italian Egg and Chicken

Cook and Prep Time: 50 <u>minutes</u> / Serves: 4 <u>servings</u>

What you need:
- 5 eggs (large)
- 1 1/2 tablespoons mustard
- 1 teaspoon garlic & herb seasoning
- 1/4 cup cream (heavy whipping)
- 1/4 cup tomato sauce
- 2 cups chicken breast, cooked & diced
- 6 ounces broccoli florets (frozen)
- 1/4 cup Parmesan cheese, grated
- 1/2 teaspoon parsley flakes
- 1/2 cup cheese (extra sharp), such as pepper jack or mozzarella, shredded

How to make it:
1. Start by preparing all the ingredients together and your Air Fryer then preheat your fryer to 325F.
2. Then in a mixing bowl, whisk the eggs then whisk in the cream, garlic & herb seasoning, and mustard.
3. After blending, gradually whisk in the tomato sauce till no longer lumpy then add the broccoli and chicken; stir to mix.
4. Next, grease a dish that will for your basket and transfer the chicken mixture into the bowl, spreading to an even layer.
5. Lastly, sprinkle the parmesan and parsley on top, pressing to adhere then place the dish in the basket; cook for 24-32

minutes or till the top is crust-like and top with the extra-sharp cheese.
6. **Serve and enjoy!**

Desserts, Snacks And Appetizers

Chocolate and Banana Sandwich

Cook and Prep Time: 8 <u>minutes</u> / Serves: 2 <u>servings</u>

What you need:
- Butter softened
- 4 slices of white bread
- ¼ cup chocolate hazelnut spread Nutella
- 1 banana

How to make it:
1. Start by preparing all the ingredients together and your Air Fryer then pre-heat the air fryer to 370ºF.
2. Then spread the softened butter on one side of all the slices of bread and place the slices, buttered side down on the counter.
3. Next, spread the chocolate hazelnut spread on the other side of the bread slices.
4. After that, cut the banana in half and then slice each half into three slices lengthwise and place the banana slices on two slices of bread and top with the remaining slices of bread to make two sandwiches.
5. Next, cut the sandwiches in half this will help them all fit in the air fryer at once then transfer the sandwiches to the air fryer.
6. Lastly, air-fry at 370ºF for 5 minutes then flip the sandwiches over and air-fry for another 2 to 3 minutes, or until the top bread slices are nicely browned.

Serve and enjoy!

My Version of Molten Lava Cake

Cook and Prep Time: 15 <u>minutes</u> / Serves: 4 <u>servings</u>

What you need:
- 1.5 tbsp. Self-Rising Flour
- 3.5 tbsp. Baker's Sugar, not powdered
- 3.5 oz. Unsalted Butter
- 3.5 oz. Dark Chocolate, chopped
- 2 Eggs

How to make it:
1. Start by preparing all the ingredients together and your Air Fryer then grease and flour 4 standard oven-safe ramekins.
2. After that, melt dark chocolate and butter in a microwave-safe bowl on level 7 for 3 minutes, stirring throughout and remove from microwave and stir until even consistency.
3. Next, beat the eggs and sugar until pale and frothy and pour the melted chocolate mixture into egg mixture then stir in the flour and mix well.
4. After that, fill the ramekins about 3/4 full with cake mixture and bake in the preheated air fryer at 375 degrees for 10 minutes.
5. Lastly, remove from the air fryer and allow it to cool in a ramekin for 2 minutes. Gradually turn ramekins upside down onto serving plate, tapping the bottom with a butter knife to loosen edges.
6. Drizzle with any syrup.

Serve and enjoy!

Heart-Shaped Cookies

Cook and Prep Time: 25 minutes / Serves: 2 servings
What you need:
- Heart-Shaped Cutter
- 250 g Plain Flour
- 75 g Caster Sugar
- 175 g Butter
- 1 tsp. Vanilla Essence
- Chocolate Buttons

How to make it:
1. Start by preparing all the ingredients together and your Air Fryer then preheat the air fryer to 180c.
2. Get a mixing bowl place all your ingredients apart from your chocolate and rub the fat into the other ingredients to create a dough.
3. When the dough is big enough as a ball. roll it out and cut it into heart shapes with your cutter.
4. Then place it into the air fryer on top of a baking sheet with a little gap in between each one and cook for 10 minutes on 180c.
5. Next, open the air fryer and place the chocolate buttons into the top of the half-baked dough.
6. Lastly, cook for a further 10 minutes on 160c.

Serve and enjoy!

Sweet Dough Dippers with Chocolate Sauce

Cook and Prep Time: 30 minutes / Serves: 10 servings

What you need:
- 1 pound bread dough, defrosted
- ½ cup of butter melted

- 1 cup of sugar
- 1 cup heavy cream
- 12 oz. semi-sweet chocolate chips
- 2 tbsp. Amaretto liqueur or almond extract

How to make it:
1. Start by preparing all the ingredients together and your Air Fryer then pre-heat the air fryer to 350ºF.
2. Then roll the dough into two 15-inch logs and cut each log into 20 slices.
3. After that, cut each slice in half and twist the dough halves together 3 to 4 times and place the twisted dough on a cookie sheet, brush with melted butter and sprinkle sugar over the dough twists.
4. Then brush the bottom of the air fryer basket with melted butter and air-fry the dough twists in batches; place 8 to 12 in the air fryer basket.
5. Next, air-fry for 5 minutes then turn the dough strips over and brush the other side with butter and air-fry for an additional 3 minutes.
6. Meanwhile, make the chocolate amaretto sauce. Bring the heavy cream to a simmer over medium heat.
7. Place the chocolate chips in a large bowl and pour the hot cream over the chocolate chips. Stir until the chocolate starts to melt then switch to a wire whisk and whisk until the chocolate is completely melted and the sauce is smooth.
8. Stir in the Amaretto then transfer to a serving dish.
9. When dough twists are complete, place them into a shallow dish and brush with melted butter and generously coat with sugar, shaking the dish to cover both sides.
10. **Lastly, serve the sugared dough dippers with the warm chocolate Amaretto sauce on the side.**

11. # Enjoy!

Air-Fried Classic Apple Pie

Cook and Prep Time: 40 <u>minutes</u> / Serves: 8 <u>servings</u>

What you need:
- 1 pie crust
- Baking spray
- 1 large apple, chopped
- 2 teaspoons lemon juice
- 1 tablespoon ground cinnamon
- 2 tablespoon sugar
- ½ teaspoon vanilla extract
- 1 tablespoon butter
- 1 beaten egg
- 1 tablespoon raw sugar

How to make it:
1. Start by preparing all the ingredients together and your Air Fryer then defrost pre-made pie crust according to package directions.
2. After that, pre-heat the Air fryer on the highest degree while you are preparing the pie.
3. Use a smaller baking tin then cut 1 crust about a ⅛ of an inch larger than the tin then the second one should be a little smaller than the baking tin. You have to roll the crust a tiny bit with a rolling pin to stretch the pie crust then set the smaller one aside.
4. Next, spray the baking tin with the baking spray and place the larger cut crust into the baking pan and set aside.
5. Get a small bowl, place the chopped apple, lemon juice, cinnamon, sugar, and vanilla extract and mix to combine.
6. After that, pour the apples into the baking pan with the pie crust and top apples with pieces of butter.

7. Put the second pie crust over the top of the apples and pinch edge and make a few slits in the top of the dough.
8. Next, spread the beaten egg over the top of the crust and sprinkle raw sugar over the top of the egg mixture then place the pie in the Air Fryer basket.
9. Lastly, set the timer for 30 minutes at 320 Degrees. Let cool.
10. **Serve and enjoy!**

Classic Chocolate Cake in an Air-Fryer

Cook and Prep Time: 35 <u>minutes</u> / Serves: 4 <u>servings</u>

What you need:
- 3 eggs
- 1/2 cup sour cream
- 1 cup flour
- 2/3 cup sugar
- 1 stick butter room temperature
- 1/3 cup cocoa powder
- 1 teaspoon baking powder
- 1/2 teaspoon baking soda
- 2 teaspoons vanilla

How to make it:
1. Start by preparing all the ingredients together and your Air Fryer then preheat Air fryer to 320 degrees.
2. Mix ingredients on low and then pour into oven attachment.
3. After that, place in Air fryer basket and slide into Air fryer then set the timer to 25 minutes.
4. When the timer beeps, insert use toothpick to see if the cake is done then cool cake on a wire rack.
5. Serve with your easy chocolate frosting.

Enjoy!

Air-Fried Chocolate Frosting

Cook and Prep Time: 5 <u>minutes</u> / Serves: 4 <u>servings</u>

What you need:
- 2 cups icing powdered sugar
- 1 stick butter room temperature
- 2 tablespoons cocoa powder
- 2 tablespoons heavy cream
- 1/8 teaspoon salt

How to make it:
Start by preparing all the ingredients together then combine ingredients in mixer on low speed until well blended.

Quick and Easy Churro Donut

Cook and Prep Time: 1 hour 25 minutes / Serves: 6 servings

What you need:
- 1 cup white all-purpose flour
- 1/4 cup organic sugar
- 1 teaspoon baking powder
- 1/4 teaspoon cinnamon
- 1/2 teaspoon salt
- 2 tablespoons aquafaba
- 1 tablespoon melted coconut oil
- 1/4 cup soy or almond milk
- 2 teaspoons cinnamon
- 2 tablespoons sugar

How to make it:
2. Start by preparing all the ingredients together and your Air Fryer.
3. Get a bowl then combine the flour, sugar, baking powder, cinnamon and salt and mix well.
4. After that, add the aquafaba, coconut oil, and soy milk then mix well.
5. Next, stick the bowl of dough into the refrigerator for at least an hour.
6. Get another bowl then mix together the cinnamon and remaining 2 tablespoons of sugar then set this aside.
7. After that, cut a piece of parchment paper so it covers some of the bottoms of your air fryer. Take attention that it doesn't cover it completely.

8. Then remove the dough from the fridge, and give it a quick knead and divide it and forming the pieces into 12 balls.
9. Next, dredge each ball in cinnamon sugar, and arrange into a single layer on the parchment paper, leaving at least 1? of room around each ball.
10. Air fry at 370F for 6 minutes just remember, do not shake.
11. Lastly, let them cool for 5-10 minutes before removing from the basket.

Serve and enjoy!

Special Butter Cake

Cook and Prep Time: 40 <u>minutes</u> / Serves: 6 <u>servings</u>

What you need:
- 115g butter
- 2 eggs
- 100g castor sugar
- 100g self-rising flour, sifted
- 30ml milk
- 1tsp vanilla extract
- 1 tbsp of cocoa powder

How to make it:
1. Start by preparing all the ingredients together and your Air Fryer then preheat air fryer at 375 degrees F.
2. Line the 6" baking tin base and grease the side of the tin
3. Beat the sugar and the butter in a mixer till fluffy
4. Then add eggs one at a time and add the vanilla extract and milk. Mix well in mixer
5. Add sifted flour then incorporated all
6. Scoop half batter out then set aside
7. Add in mixer cocoa powder to the batter and mix well

8. Scoop 2 tablespoons of the plain batter in the center of the baking tin. Then scoop 2 tablespoons of chocolate batter in the center of the plain batter in the baking tin. Keep scooping by alternating both batters till finish.
9. Then every scoop of batter into the tin, try to tap the tin to let the batter spread out.

Place the baking tin in the air fryer and bake at 160C for 30 minutes or till skewer emerges cleanly.

Air-Fried Jalapeno Bites

Cook and Prep Time: 10 <u>minutes</u> / Serves: 4 <u>servings</u>

What you need:
- 10 jalapeno peppers halved and deseeded
- 8 oz. of cream cheese
- 1/4 cup fresh parsley
- 3/4 cup gluten-free tortilla or bread crumbs

How to make it:
1. Start by preparing all the ingredients together and your Air Fryer.
2. After that, mix together 1/2 of crumbs and cream cheese then stir in the parsley.
3. Next, stuff each pepper with the mixture and gently press the tops of the peppers into the remaining 1/4 c of crumbs to create the top coating.
4. Lastly, cook in an air fryer at 370 degrees F for 8 minutes.
5. Let cool.

Serve and enjoy!

Classic Snack Donuts

Cook and Prep Time: 17 minutes / Serves: 4 servings

What you need:
- 1/2 cup granulated sugar
- 1 tablespoon ground cinnamon
- 1 (16.3-ounce) can flaky large biscuits
- Olive oil spray
- 4 tablespoons unsalted butter, melted

How to make it:
1. Start by preparing all the ingredients together and your Air Fryer then line a baking sheet with parchment paper.
2. Combine sugar and cinnamon in a bowl then set aside.
3. After that, remove the biscuits from the can, separate them, and place them on the baking sheet and use a 1-inch round biscuit cutter to cut holes out of the center of each biscuit.
4. Lightly coat an air fryer basket with olive or coconut oil then place 3 to 4 donuts in a single layer in the air fryer.
5. Next, close the air fryer and set to 350°F and cook, flipping halfway through, until the donuts golden-brown for 6 minutes.
6. Transfer donuts place to the baking sheet and repeat with the remaining biscuits.
7. Lastly, brush both sides of the warm donuts with melted butter, place in the cinnamon sugar, and flip to coat both sides.

Serve and enjoy!

Easy Apple Chips

Cook and Prep Time: 13 minutes / Serves: 3 servings

What you need:
- 3 large sweet, crisp apples, such as Honeycrisp, Fuji, Jazz, or Pink Lady
- 3/4 teaspoon ground cinnamon
- a pinch of salt

How to make it:
1. Start by preparing all the ingredients together and your Air Fryer then preheat the air fryer at 390 degrees F.
2. After that, wash the apples in warm water or apple cider vinegar then core the apples.
3. Then cut the apple sideways into 1/8th-inch rounds.
4. After that, mix cinnamon and salt in a bowl.
5. Next, arrange apples in a single layer and sprinkle or rub some cinnamon and salt mixture and arrange a single layer of the above apple slices in the air fryer.
6. After that, cook for 8 minutes at 390 degrees F, flipping sides halfway through.
7. Once done, cool the chips on a cooling rack.

Serve and enjoy!

Special Sweet Potato Tots Snacks

Cook and Prep Time: 1 hour 20 minutes / Serves: 4 servings

What you need:
- 2 small sweet potatoes, peeled
- 1 tablespoon potato starch
- 1/8 teaspoon garlic powder
- 1 1/4 teaspoons kosher, divided
- 3/4 cup no-salt-added ketchup
- Cooking spray

How to make it:
1. Start by preparing all the ingredients together and your Air Fryer.

2. Then bring a pot with water to a boil over high heat and stir in the potatoes, and cook until just fork-tender, about 15 minutes.
3. After that, transfer potatoes to a plate to cool, about 15 minutes.
4. Get a bowl then grate potatoes using the large holes of a box grater.
5. Gradually toss with potato starch, garlic powder and 1 teaspoon salt. Shape mixture into about 24 (1-inch) tot-shaped cylinders.
6. Next, lightly coat air fryer basket with cooking spray then place 1/2 of tots in a single layer in the basket.
7. Lastly, cook at 400°F until lightly browned, 12 to 14 minutes, turning tots halfway through cook time and remove from fry basket and sprinkle with 1/8 teaspoon salt then repeat with remaining tots and salt.
8. Serve the tots with ketchup.

Enjoy!

Pepperoni Pizza in Whole Wheat Pita Bread

Cook and Prep Time: 10 minutes / Serves: 4 servings

What you need:
- 1 whole-wheat pita
- 2 tbsp. pizza sauce or marinara sauce
- 1/8th cup mozzarella cheese, shredded
- 1/8th cup cheddar cheese,
- 8 slices pepperoni
- olive oil spray
- 1 tbsp. chopped parsley, optional to garnish the pizza when it has cooled

How to make it:
1. Start by preparing all the ingredients together and your Air Fryer.
2. Then drizzle the sauce on top of the pita bread and load the pepperoni and shredded cheese on top.
3. After that, spray the top of the pizza with olive oil spray and place it in the Air Fryer for 8 minutes at 400 degrees F.
4. Then check in on the pizza at the 7-minute mark, to ensure it does not overcook.

After that, remove the pizza from the Air Fryer.

All-Time Favorite Banana Bread

Cook and Prep Time: 50 minutes / Serves: 4 servings

What you need:
- 3/4 cup white whole wheat flour
- 1 teaspoon cinnamon
- 1/2 teaspoon salt

- 1/4 teaspoon baking soda
- 2 medium ripe bananas, mashed
- 2 large eggs, lightly beaten
- 1/2 cup granulated sugar
- 1/3 cup plain non-fat yogurt
- 2 tablespoons vegetable oil
- 1 teaspoon Vanilla extract
- 2 tablespoons toasted walnuts, roughly chopped
- Cooking spray

How to make it:
1. Start by preparing all the ingredients together and your Air Fryer.
2. Then after that, line the bottom of a 6-inch round cake pan with parchment paper; lightly coat pan with cooking spray.
3. Mix together the flour, cinnamon, salt and baking soda in a bowl then set aside.
4. Get another bowl and whisk together mashed bananas, eggs, sugar, yogurt, oil and vanilla. Gently stir wet ingredients into flour mixture until well combined.
5. After that, pour batter into prepared pan and sprinkle with walnuts.
6. Next, heat a 5.3-qt air fryer to 310°F and then place the pan in an air fryer and cook until browned and a wooden pick inserted in the middle comes out clean for 35 minutes, turning the pan halfway through cook time.
7. Lastly, transfer bread to a wire rack to cool in the pan for 15 minutes before turning out and slicing.

Serve and enjoy!

Air-Fried Keto Avocado Fries

Cook and Prep Time: 30 minutes / Serves: 4 servings

What you need:

- 1/2 cup all-purpose flour
- 1 1/2 teaspoons black pepper
- 2 large eggs
- 1 tablespoon water
- 1/2 cup bread crumbs (I use Panko)
- 2 avocados, cut into 8 wedges each
- Cooking spray
- 1/4 teaspoon salt
- 1/4 cup no-salt-added ketchup
- 2 tablespoons canola mayonnaise
- 1 tablespoon apple cider vinegar
- 1 tablespoon Sriracha chili sauce

How to make it:
1. Start by preparing all the ingredients together and your Air Fryer.
2. Get a shallow dish then combine the flour and pepper together.
3. After that, lightly beat eggs and water in a second dish then place panko in a third dish.
4. Next, dredge avocado wedges in flour, shaking off excess then dip in egg mixture, allowing any excess to drip off.
5. After that, dredge in panko, pressing to adhere and coat the avocado wedges well with cooking spray.
6. Then place avocado wedges in the air fryer basket, and cook 7 to 8 minutes at 400°F until golden.
7. Then turning avocado wedges over halfway through cooking and remove from air fryer; sprinkle with salt.
8. Meanwhile, whisk together ketchup, mayonnaise, vinegar, and Sriracha in a bowl to create the sauce.
9. Serve the fries with the sauce.

10. Enjoy!

Low Carb Dessert Pudding

Cook and Prep Time: 50 <u>minutes</u> / Serves: 2 <u>servings</u>

What you need:
- 1 lemon, zest only
- 1/4 cup blackberries
- 1/4 cup coconut flour
- 1/4 teaspoon baking powder
- 10 drops liquid stevia
- 2 tablespoon butter
- 2 tablespoon coconut oil
- 2 tablespoon erythritol
- 2 tablespoon heavy cream
- 2 teaspoon lemon juice
- 5 egg yolks

How to make it:
1. Start by preparing all the ingredients together and your Air Fryer then preheat the fryer to 325F.
2. After that, separate the whites and the yolks of the eggs and measure all the dry ingredients.
3. Then measure also the coconut oil and butter.
4. Next, whisk the egg yolks till the color turns pale then add the stevia and the erythritol; whisk till combined.
5. After that, sift the dry ingredients into the wet ingredients; mix well and divide the mixture between 2 ramekins.
6. Lastly, push 2 tablespoons of blackberries into each ramekin, slightly crushing them before adding to the batter and put the ramekin in the basket; cook for 16 to 20 minutes.

Serve and enjoy!

Yummy Cream Cheesecake with Vanilla

Cook and Prep Time: 20 <u>minutes</u> / Serves: 9 <u>servings</u>

What you need:
- 1 ounces erythritol
- 1 teaspoon vanilla extract
- 1/2 cup heavy cream
- 4 1/2 ounces cream cheese, softened

How to make it:
1. Start by preparing all the ingredients together and your Air Fryer.
2. And then mix the erythritol, vanilla, and cream cheese in your kitchen aid or into a mixing bowl and use a hand mixer for 2 minutes using low speed till smooth.
3. After that, stir in half of the cream then mix for 2 minutes and let sit for 3 to 5 minutes to give the erythritol enough time to dissolve.
4. Next, add the rest of the cream; mix for 3 minutes using medium speed until thickened and firm peaks appear.
5. Slowly, transfer the mixture into a piping bag; pipe into mini cupcake liners then refrigerate for at least 1 hour.

Serve and enjoy!

Keto Crispy Bacon Burger

Cook and Prep Time: 50 minutes / Serves: 6 servings

What you need:
- 6 cubes cheddar cheese, smoked
- 6 rounds sausage patties, raw
- 6 slices bacon
- Cumin
- Pepper
- Powdered onion
- Salt

How to make it:
1. Start by preparing all the ingredients together and your Air Fryer then preheat the fryer t0 325F.

2. After then, put the sausage into a sheet of parchment paper smaller than the basket area to allow air to flow through and season with the pepper, salt, powdered onion, and cumin.
3. Next, put at least 1 cube of cheese in the center of the sausage roll the sausage to cover the cheese and form into a ball between your palms then gently, wrap each ball with the bacon.
4. Lastly, place parchment in the basket; cook for 48 minutes. Serve and enjoy!

Healthy Snack Bars

Cook and Prep Time: 50 minutes / Serves: 6 servings

What you need:
- 1 cup pecan halves
- 1/2 cup almond flour
- 1/4 cup coconut oil
- 1/4 cup golden flaxseed meal
- 1/4 cup shredded unsweetened coconut
- 1/8 cup maple syrup
- 1/8 teaspoon liquid stevia

How to make it:
1. Start by preparing all the ingredients together and your Air Fryer.
2. After then, toast the pecans in your air fryer for 7 minutes while shaking occasionally then let them cool.
3. Next, transfer them to some plastic bag; crush using your rolling pin then put the pecans and the rest of the dry ingredients in a bowl; mix well.
4. Stir in the wet ingredients and mix till it forms a crumbly dough.
5. Next, press the mixture into a 5 1/2x3 1/2 baking pan or similar that fits in your fryer.
6. Lastly, cook at 325F for 16 to 20 minutes and remove and let completely cool then refrigerate for at least an hour.

7. Slice then serve.
Enjoy!

Guacamole Different Ways

Cook and Prep Time: 35 minutes / Serves: 3 servings

What you need:
- 1 tablespoon roasted garlic
- 1/2 lime, juice only
- 1/3 bell pepper medium, red, chopped
- 1/3 cup cilantro, chopped
- 1/4 small onion
- 2 medium avocados
- 4 slices bacon
- Salt and pepper

How to make it:
1. Start by preparing all the ingredients together and your Air Fryer.
2. After that, cook the bacon in your fryer then crumble the cooked bacon and set aside and keep the bacon fat.
3. Next, slice the avocado, remove the seeds and pits then transfer the avocado meat to a bowl and stir in the garlic, cilantro, and bell pepper.
4. Lastly, add the crumbled bacon and bacon fat; mix well then add pepper and salt to season and lime juice then mix well.

Serve and enjoy!

Mozzarella Pizza Chips

Cook and Prep Time: 25 minutes / Serves: 10 servings

What you need:

- 2 1/1 ounces mozzarella cheese, shredded
- 3 ounces pepperoni, sliced

How to make it:
1. Start by preparing all the ingredients together and your Air Fryer then preheat your fryer to 370F.
2. After that, place a single layer of pepperoni in the basket and cook for 4 minutes or till they are semi-crisp and the fat is rendered.
3. Next, sprinkle the cheese on top; cook for 2-3 minutes more or till the cheese is melted and slightly crisp.
4. Lastly, transfer to paper towels to drain excess grease; let cool for 3 to 4 minutes to crisp them even more.
5. You can serve with the marinara sauce.

Enjoy!

Low Carb Beef Taco Tartlets

Cook and Prep Time: 60 <u>minutes</u> / Serves: 11 <u>servings</u>

What you need:
  For the pastry:
- 5 tablespoons cold butter
- 3 tablespoons coconut flour
- 2 tablespoons of ice water
- 1/4 teaspoon salt
- 1/4 teaspoon paprika
- 1/4 teaspoon cayenne
- 1 teaspoon xanthan gum
- 1 teaspoon oregano
- 1 cup almond flour, blanched

  For the Filling:
- 1 tablespoon olive oil

- 1 teaspoon cumin
- 1 teaspoon salt
- 1 teaspoon Worcestershire
- 1/2 teaspoon pepper
- 1/3 cup cheese
- 1/4 teaspoon cinnamon
- 2 tablespoons tomato paste
- 2 teaspoons garlic, minced
- 2 teaspoons yellow mustard
- 3 green onion stalks, chopped
- 400 grams ground beef
- 80 grams mushroom, sliced

How to make it:
1. Start by preparing all the ingredients together and your Air Fryer then preheat the fryer to 305F and mix all the dry ingredients and transfer to your food processor.
2. After that, chop the cold butter and add in the processor then pulse till a crumbly dough forms, adding 1 tablespoon ice water as needed to achieve the correct consistency; freeze for 10 minutes to chill.
3. Next, place the dough between pieces of Silpat or non-stick baking mat and roll to thin.
4. Then cut small circles of dough using a glass or a cookie cutter and place each dough circle in the bottom paper lined tin muffin cups.
5. Meanwhile, prepare the mushrooms, garlic, and spring onion then sauté the garlic and spring onion with the olive oil in a pan.
6. Stir in the beef; add the Worcestershire and spices; sauté till seared and add the mushroom; stir to mix and sauté till well brown.
7. Next, add the mustard and tomato paste and mix well.
8. After that, evenly divide and spoon the beef mixture into the tartlets and sprinkle the cheese on top.

9. Lastly, cook the tartlets for 16 to 20 minutes then remove from the basket, let completely cool, and remove the liners from the muffin cups; peel the liners from the tartlets.
Serve and enjoy!

Air-Fried Corndog Muffins

Cook and Prep Time: 40 minutes / Serves: 20 servings

What you need:
- 1 egg
- 1 tablespoon powdered psyllium husk
- 1/2 cup almond flour, blanched
- 1/2 cup flaxseed meal
- 1/3 cup sour cream
- 1/4 cup butter, melted
- 1/4 cup coconut milk
- 1/4 teaspoon baking powder
- 1/4 teaspoon salt
- 3 hot dogs
- 3 tablespoons Swerve sweetener

How to make it:
1. Start by preparing all the ingredients together and your Air Fryer then preheat your fryer to 350F.
2. After that, mix every dry ingredient till well blended.
3. Stir in the butter, coconut milk, sour cream, and egg; mix well then grease well 20 mini silicone muffin cups.
4. Then divide the batter between them and slice the hotdogs crosswise into halves. Insert each half in the center of each muffin.
5. Next, cook the muffins for 12 minutes or till the tops are light brown then push the hotdogs that rose back into the muffin.

6. Lastly, transfer and let cool slightly before removing to a cooling rack.

Serve and enjoy!

Homemade BLT Dip

Cook and Prep Time: 40 <u>minutes</u> / Serves: 20 <u>servings</u>

What you need:
- 1/2 cup mayonnaise
- 1/2 cup sour cream
- 1/2 slicing tomato
- 2 tablespoons fresh chives, chopped
- 3/4 cups cheddar cheese, shredded
- 4 ounces cream cheese, softened
- 6 ounces bacon

How to make it:
1. Start by preparing all the ingredients together and your Air Fryer.
2. After that, cook the bacon in your fryer and remove it from the basket.
3. Get a bowl then add the sour cream, mayonnaise, and cream cheese; stir till well mixed then crumble the bacon; add to the cheese mixture, stirring to mix.
4. Then add the cheddar cheese, saving some for topping and dice the tomato and save for topping, and add the rest to the dip.
5. Next, spread the mixture into a heatproof container that will fit your fryer.
6. Lastly, top with the reserved cheese and tomato and cook at 350F for 16 minutes or till bubbly and hot.
7. Serve with chives on top.

Enjoy!

Keto Crispy Onion Rings with Sauce

Cook and Prep Time: 35 minutes / Serves: 4 servings

What you need:
- 1 cup parmesan cheese
- 1 egg
- 1 tablespoon ketchup
- 1 tablespoon water
- 1 teaspoon Dijon mustard
- 1 teaspoon smoked paprika
- 1/2 cup arrowroot flour
- 1/2 teaspoon salt, divided
- 1/4 cup plain Greek yogurt
- 1/4 teaspoon powdered garlic
- 1/4 teaspoon paprika
- 1 pc. 10 ounces sweet onion, sliced into 1/2-inch-thick rounds & rings separated
- 2 tablespoons mayonnaise
- Cooking spray

How to make it:
1. Start by preparing all the ingredients together and your Air Fryer.
2. Get a dish then mix 1/4 teaspoon salt, smoked paprika, and flour.
3. Get another dish then lightly whisk the egg with water.
4. Get a third dish then stir the parmesan cheese and rest of the salt.
5. After that, start dredging the rings in the flour mix; shake excess off then dip in the egg mix; let the excess drip off.

6. Then dredge in the parmesan mix; press to adhere well. Spray with the cooking spray well on both sides.
7. Arrange them in a single layer, place some onion rings on the air fryer basket and cook for 10 minutes at 375F or till both sides are crispy and golden brown, turning halfway through.
8. After that, transfer to a platter; cover and keep warm while the rest of the rings cook.
9. Next, mix the paprika, powdered garlic, mustard, ketchup, mayonnaise, and yogurt in a bowl till smooth.
10. Lastly, arrange 6 rings on each plate and scoop 2 tablespoons of sauce on the side of the onions.
11. **Serve and enjoy!**

Healthy Keto Beet Chips

Cook and Prep Time: 45 <u>minutes</u> / Serves: 4 <u>servings</u>

-

What you need:
- 1/4 teaspoon black pepper
- 2 teaspoons canola oil
- 3 red beets (medium, around 1 1/2 pounds), peeled & into 1/8-inch-thick pieces (around 3 cups)
- 3/4 teaspoon salt

How to make it:
1. Start by preparing all the ingredients together and your Air Fryer.
2. Get a bowl then mix the beets with pepper, salt, and oil.
3. After that, put 1/2 of the slices in the basket; cook for 25 to 30 minutes at 320F or till crisp and dry, shaking every 5 minutes.
4. Then repeat the procedure with your remaining slices.

Serve and enjoy!

Cinnamon Apple Chips with Yogurt Almond Dip

Cook and Prep Time: 25 minutes / Serves: 4 servings

What you need:
- 1 tablespoon almond butter
- 1 teaspoon erythritol
- 1 teaspoon ground cinnamon
- 1/4 cup plain Greek yogurt
- 2 teaspoons canola oil
- 1 pc 8 ounces apple
- Cooking spray

How to make it:
1. Start by preparing all the ingredients together and your Air Fryer.
2. Then prepare and slice the apple into thin pieces using a mandolin.
3. After that, put the slices in a bowl and add the oil and cinnamon; toss to evenly coat.
4. Grease the basket with the cooking spray.
5. Next, in a single layer, put 7 slices in it; cook for 12 minutes at 375F, flipping every 4 minutes and keeping them flattened in the basket.
6. Lastly, transfer to a plate then continue with the repeat the procedure with your remaining slices.

Serve and enjoy!

Super Healthy Kale Chips

Cook and Prep Time: 30 minutes / Serves: 2 servings

What you need:
- 1 tablespoon olive oil
- 1 teaspoon coconut aminos
- 1 teaspoon sesame seeds
- 1/2 teaspoon dried garlic, minced

- 1/4 teaspoon poppy seeds
- 6 packed cups kale leaves, torn, stems & ribs removed

How to make it:
1. Start by preparing all the ingredients together and your Air Fryer then wash the kale leaves and let them dry completely.
2. After that, tear them in 1 1/2-inch piece and put in a bowl then add the coconut aminos and olive oil; toss to coat, rubbing them gently in the process.
3. Then put 1/3 of the leaves in the basket; cook for 6 minutes at 375F, shaking halfway through.
4. Next, transfer to a baking sheet and sprinkle with the poppy seeds, garlic, and sesame seeds evenly right away.
5. Lastly, repeat with the rest of the leaves.

Serve and enjoy!

Air-Fried Pretzel Recipe

Cook and Prep Time: 40 minutes / Serves: 6 servings

What you need:
- 3/4 cup almond flour
- 2 tablespoons cream cheese
- 1/2 tablespoon pretzel salt
- 1 teaspoon xanthan gum
- 1 teaspoon dried yeast, around 1/2 sachet
- 1 tablespoon warm water
- 1 tablespoon butter, melted
- 1 eggs room temperature
- 1 1/2 cups mozzarella cheese, shredded

How to make it:
1. Start by preparing all the ingredients together and your Air Fryer.
2. After that, put the cream cheese and mozzarella cheese in a microwave-safe bowl.

3. Microwave for 30 seconds till completely melted and almost liquid, stirring every period then mix the yeast with the warm water till completely dissolve; let sit for 2 minutes to activate.
4. Next, attach the dough hook in your stand mixer and place the xanthan gum and almond meal; mix well.
5. Then add 1 tablespoon melted butter, yeast mixture, and eggs; mix well and stir in the melted cheeses; knead for 5 to 10 minutes or till well incorporated.
6. Next, divide the dough into 6 portions and roll each ball into skinny, long legs.
7. Then twist each into pretzel shapes and line the basket with parchment paper smaller than its area to allow air to flow through.
8. After that, place 1-2 pretzels in the basket, leaving a little space between each piece for rising and brush the tops with butter and season with the salt.
9. Lastly, cook at 365-370F for 9-12 minutes or till golden brown and repeat with the rest of the pretzels.

Serve and enjoy!

Movie Cheesy Popcorn Puffs

Cook and Prep Time: 10 minutes / Serves: 4 servings

What you need:
- 4 ounces cheddar cheese

How to make it:
1. Start by preparing all the ingredients together and your Air Fryer then preheat the fryer to 365-370F.
2. After that, prepare this recipe 24 hours before cooking and slice the cheddar into 1/4-inch cubes then put them in a parchment paper-lined sheet pan.

3. Next, cover with a clean dish or tea towel then leave for 24 hours to dry out or longer as needed if you live in a humid area.
4. Then create a parchment paper container smaller than the basket area to allow air to flow through.
5. After that, place the cheese in the paper container and put it in the basket.
6. Lastly cook for 3 to 4 minutes or till puffed and transfer and let stand for 10 minutes to cool before serving.

Serve and enjoy!

Crunchy Cheesy Broccoli Snack

Cook and Prep Time: 10 minutes / Serves: 1 serving

What you need:
- 1 tablespoon olive oil
- 1 tablespoon parmesan cheese grated
- 1/3 broccoli
- 1/3 tablespoon butter, melted
- Pinch pepper
- Pinch salt

How to make it:
1. Start by preparing all the ingredients together and your Air Fryer then preheat the fryer to 365-370F.
2. After that, slice the broccoli into evenly-sized pieces then get a bowl and put them.
3. Then add the pepper, salt, parmesan, melted butter, and oil and mix using clean hands and ensure each floret is coated with the other ingredients.
4. Next, spread the broccoli in the basket.
5. Lastly, cook for 16-20 minutes, flipping halfway through.

Serve and enjoy!

Air-Fried Mushroom Fries

Cook and Prep Time: 38 <u>minutes</u> / Serves: 2 <u>servings</u>

What you need:
- 1 egg, whisked
- 1 tablespoon dry chives, for garnishing
- 1/2 cup Parmesan cheese, shredded
- 1/2 teaspoon smoked paprika
- 1/2 teaspoon powdered garlic
- 1/4 cup cheddar cheese, shredded
- 1/4 teaspoon cayenne pepper
- 2 Portobello mushroom
- 3 bacon strips

How to make it:
1. Start by preparing all the ingredients together and your Air Fryer then cook your bacon pieces in the fryer till crisp.
2. After that, transfer and let cool before crumbling or slicing then slice the mushrooms into 1/4-inch thick pieces.
3. Slice the ends at an angle into French fry tips than in a food processor, blend the parmesan with the seasoning till well mixed.
4. After that, transfer to a bowl then whisk the egg in a bowl.
5. Next, dip the mushroom pieces in the egg, shaking excess off then roll in the parmesan mixture, pressing to adhere.
6. After that, set the fryer to 400F then spray the basket with cooking spray.
7. Next, spread an even layer of mushroom fries in the foil. Bake for 8 minutes and create a foil container smaller than the basket area to allow air to flow through.
8. Lastly, transfer the mushroom fries to the foil container then sprinkle the top with the cheddar and bacon and fry till the cheese melts.

9. Serve top with chives.
Enjoy!

Air-Fried Healthy Pesto Keto Crackers

Cook and Prep Time: 35 minutes / Serves: 3 servings

What you need:
- 1 1/2 tablespoons butter
- 1 tablespoon basil pesto
- 1/2 & 1/8 cups almond flour
- 1/2 clove garlic, pressed
- 1/4 teaspoon baking powder
- 1/4 teaspoon salt
- 1/8 teaspoon dried basil
- 1/8 teaspoon ground black pepper
- Small pinch cayenne pepper

How to make it:
1. Start by preparing all the ingredients together and your Air Fryer then preheat your fryer to 305F.
2. After that, create a parchment paper container smaller than the basket area to allow air to flow through.
3. Get a bowl then mix the baking powder, pepper, salt, and flour till smooth and stir in the garlic, cayenne, and basil; stir till evenly incorporated.
4. Add the pesto; mix till the mixture forms a dough then place the dough between sheets of parchment paper.
5. After that, flatten it into an even 1 1/2 –mm thickness then cut into size/sizes that will fit your paper container or into desired shapes.
6. Next, put a single layer of cracker dough in the paper container and place the paper container in the basket.
7. Lastly, cook for 11-14 minutes or till light brown, flipping halfway through then transfer.

Serve and enjoy!

Low Carb Chia Seeds Crackers

Cook and Prep Time: 55 minutes / Serves: 18 servings

What you need:
- 1 1/2 ounces cheddar cheese, shredded
- 1 tablespoon olive oil
- 1 tablespoon powdered psyllium husk
- 1/2 & 1/8 cups ice water
- 1/4 cup ground chia seeds
- 1/8 teaspoon powdered onion
- 1/8 teaspoon oregano
- 1/8 teaspoon paprika
- 1/8 teaspoon pepper
- 1/8 teaspoon powdered garlic
- 1/8 teaspoon salt
- 1/8 teaspoon xanthan gum

How to make it:
1. Start by preparing all the ingredients together and your Air Fryer then preheat the fryer to 350F.
2. After that, grind the chia seeds in your spice grinder and transfer for a bowl.
3. Then add the rest of the dry ingredients and stir in the olive oil and mix till the consistency is like wet sand.
4. Next, pour in the water; mix till very well incorporated and the mixture forms a solid dough – this might take a while since the psyllium and chia seeds absorb water gradually.
5. After that, add the cheddar, mix well using clean hands and transfer to a Silpat and leave for 5 minutes.
6. After then roll or spread the dough into 1/2 the size of the Silpat and create a parchment paper container smaller than the basket area to allow air to flow through.

7. Next, slice into sizes that will fit your paper container or desired shapes.
8. Lastly, place the paper container with a single layer of cracker dough in the basket and cook for 28-34 minutes or till crisp, turning halfway through; let cool.

Serve and enjoy!

Air-Fried Spiced Deviled Eggs with Bacon

Cook and Prep Time: 45 minutes / Serves: 3 servings

What you need:
- 1 tablespoon bacon fat, rendered
- 1 teaspoon Dijon mustard
- 1/2 teaspoon rosemary
- 1/4 cup mayonnaise
- 1/4 teaspoon cayenne pepper
- 2 bacon slices
- 5 eggs, hard-boiled

How to make it:
1. Start by preparing all the ingredients together and your Air Fryer then boil your eggs in the fryer
2. Peel the eggs once hard-boiled then set aside.
3. After that, cook the bacon in your fryer.
4. Then transfer to a paper towel and let cool to crisp more if desired and save the drippings.
5. Crumble them once cool enough to handle and slice the eggs lengthwise into halves.
6. Next, transfer the yolk to a bowl and add 1/2 of the rosemary, bacon fat, cayenne, mustard, and mayonnaise; mix well.
7. After that, sprinkle some crumbled bacon in the bottom of the egg whites.
8. Spoon your yolk mixture between your egg whites then divides the crumbled bacon on top and garnish with rosemary.

Serve and enjoy!

Keto Double Cheeseburger

Cook and Prep Time: 20 minutes / Serves: 2 servings

What you need:
- 1 pinch fresh ground black pepper
- 1 pinch powdered onion
- 1 pinch salt
- 1/2 pound ground beef
- 2 slices of preferred cheese

How to make it:
1. Start by preparing all the ingredients together and your Air Fryer.
2. After that, start forming the ground beef into 1/4 pound patties.
3. Then lightly season them with powdered onion, pepper, and salt and put the patties in the basket; cook for 12 minutes at 370F, flipping halfway through.
4. Next, when the cooking process is done, place the cheese on top of each patty.
5. Lastly, close the fryer and let stand for 1 minute to melt the cheese.

Serve and enjoy!

Chia Seed Butter Snack

Cook and Prep Time: 35 minutes / Serves: 6 servings

What you need:
- 1 1/3 tablespoons butter, melted
- 1 1/3 tablespoons erythritol, powdered
- 1 egg
- 1 tablespoon heavy cream

- 1 tablespoon Salted Caramel
- 1/3 teaspoon baking powder
- 1/6 cup chia seeds, ground
- 3/4 cup pecans, roasted
- 3-4 drops liquid stevia
- Small pinch salt

How to make it:
1. Start by preparing all the ingredients together and your Air Fryer then preheat your air fryer to 325F.
2. After that, spread the pecans in the basket and cook for 10 minutes or till the aroma is nutty.
3. Meanwhile, grind the chia seeds using your spice grinder till the texture is mealy then grind the erythritol using your spice grinder till powdered.
4. Get a bowl then mix the ground chia and powdered sweetener.
5. Next, process 2/3 of the pecans into nut butter and add the pecan butter, salt, stevia, and egg into the bowl with the erythritol and chia; stir to mix well.
6. After that, add the heavy cream, baking powder, salted caramel, and melted butter; stir to mix well then chop the rest of the pecans; add to the batter; stir to mix.
7. Lastly, transfer the mixture to a 3x3-inch baking container or similar that will fit your basket and cook for 16 minutes; let cool and slice into 6 squares.

Serve and enjoy!

Keto Blueberry Lime Cake

Cook and Prep Time: 60 <u>minutes</u> / Serves: 1 <u>serving</u>

What you need:
- 1 tablespoon coconut flour
- 1 tablespoon salted butter
- 1 teaspoon blueberry extract
- 1/2 cup almond flour
- 1/2 teaspoon baking powder
- 1/8 cup blueberries
- 1/8 cup cream cheese
- 1/8 cup erythritol
- 1/8 teaspoon liquid stevia
- 3 eggs, separated
- Juice 1/2 lime
- Zest 1/2 lime

How to make it:
1. Start by preparing all the ingredients together and your Air Fryer then preheat the fryer to 305F.
2. After that, separate egg yolks from the whites then mix all of the ingredients. Whisk the egg yolks till the color is pale. Add the cream cheese, butter, blueberry extract, liquid stevia, and the erythritol; beat till smooth.
3. Next, add the lime juice and zest; saving 1 teaspoon of the juice and whisk till smooth.
4. Then sift the dry ingredients into the wet mixture; mix well then beat the egg whites with the 1 teaspoon lime juice till stiff peaks appear and fold the egg whites into the yolk mixture.
5. Next, pour the batter into a cake or loaf pan that fits your basket.

6. Lastly, top with the berries then put the pan in the basket; cook for 28 to 32 minutes or till a toothpick comes out clean when inserted in the center.

Serve and enjoy!

Air-Fried Strawberry Shortcakes

Cook and Prep Time: 30 minutes / Serves: 3 servings

What you need:
   For the Puff cakes:

- 1 1/2 ounces cream cheese
- 1 tablespoon erythritol
- 1/4 teaspoon vanilla extract
- 1/8 teaspoon baking powder
- 2 eggs

   For the Filling:

- 1/2 cup heavy cream
- 5 medium strawberries

How to make it:
1. Start by preparing all the ingredients together and your Air Fryer then preheat the fryer to 280F.
2. After that, separate the egg yolks from the whites then whisk the egg whites till fluffy.
3. In the bowl with the egg yolks, add the erythritol, baking powder, vanilla, and cream cheese then beat till smooth.
4. Next, fold the egg whites into the yolk mixture and spread the mixture into a parchment paper container smaller than the basket area to allow air to flow through.
5. After then, create a parchment paper container smaller than the basket area to allow air to flow through and put the paper on the basket.
6. Lastly, scoop batter into the paper, making round portions; cook for 20 to 24 minutes then let cool and sandwich whipped heavy cream and strawberries between 2 cakes.
7. Serve and enjoy!

www.ingramcontent.com/pod-product-compliance
Lightning Source LLC
Chambersburg PA
CBHW072010070526
44583CB00015B/1414